CN-1   CERTIFIED NURSE EXAMINATION SERIES

This is your
PASSBOOK for...

Adult Nurse Practitioner

Test Preparation Study Guide
Questions & Answers

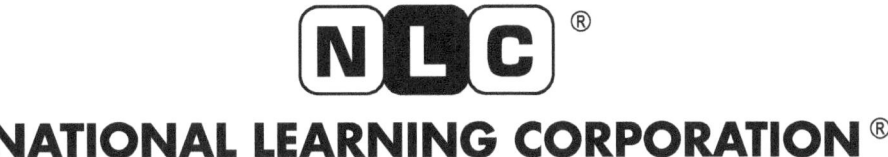

COPYRIGHT NOTICE

This book is SOLELY intended for, is sold ONLY to, and its use is RESTRICTED to individual, bona fide applicants or candidates who qualify by virtue of having seriously filed applications for appropriate license, certificate, professional and/or promotional advancement, higher school matriculation, scholarship, or other legitimate requirements of education and/or governmental authorities.

This book is NOT intended for use, class instruction, tutoring, training, duplication, copying, reprinting, excerption, or adaptation, etc., by:

1) Other publishers
2) Proprietors and/or Instructors of "Coaching" and/or Preparatory Courses
3) Personnel and/or Training Divisions of commercial, industrial, and governmental organizations
4) Schools, colleges, or universities and/or their departments and staffs, including teachers and other personnel
5) Testing Agencies or Bureaus
6) Study groups which seek by the purchase of a single volume to copy and/or duplicate and/or adapt this material for use by the group as a whole without having purchased individual volumes for each of the members of the group
7) Et al.

Such persons would be in violation of appropriate Federal and State statutes.

PROVISION OF LICENSING AGREEMENTS – Recognized educational, commercial, industrial, and governmental institutions and organizations, and others legitimately engaged in educational pursuits, including training, testing, and measurement activities, may address request for a licensing agreement to the copyright owners, who will determine whether, and under what conditions, including fees and charges, the materials in this book may be used them. In other words, a licensing facility exists for the legitimate use of the material in this book on other than an individual basis. However, it is asseverated and affirmed here that the material in this book CANNOT be used without the receipt of the express permission of such a licensing agreement from the Publishers. Inquiries re licensing should be addressed to the company, attention rights and permissions department.

All rights reserved, including the right of reproduction in whole or in part, in any form or by any means, electronic or mechanical, including photocopying, recording, or by any information storage and retrieval system, without permission in writing from the Publisher.

Copyright © 2025 by
National Learning Corporation

212 Michael Drive, Syosset, NY 11791
(516) 921-8888 • www.passbooks.com
E-mail: info@passbooks.com

PASSBOOK® SERIES

THE *PASSBOOK® SERIES* has been created to prepare applicants and candidates for the ultimate academic battlefield – the examination room.

At some time in our lives, each and every one of us may be required to take an examination – for validation, matriculation, admission, qualification, registration, certification, or licensure.

Based on the assumption that every applicant or candidate has met the basic formal educational standards, has taken the required number of courses, and read the necessary texts, the *PASSBOOK® SERIES* furnishes the one special preparation which may assure passing with confidence, instead of failing with insecurity. Examination questions – together with answers – are furnished as the basic vehicle for study so that the mysteries of the examination and its compounding difficulties may be eliminated or diminished by a sure method.

This book is meant to help you pass your examination provided that you qualify and are serious in your objective.

The entire field is reviewed through the huge store of content information which is succinctly presented through a provocative and challenging approach – the question-and-answer method.

A climate of success is established by furnishing the correct answers at the end of each test.

You soon learn to recognize types of questions, forms of questions, and patterns of questioning. You may even begin to anticipate expected outcomes.

You perceive that many questions are repeated or adapted so that you can gain acute insights, which may enable you to score many sure points.

You learn how to confront new questions, or types of questions, and to attack them confidently and work out the correct answers.

You note objectives and emphases, and recognize pitfalls and dangers, so that you may make positive educational adjustments.

Moreover, you are kept fully informed in relation to new concepts, methods, practices, and directions in the field.

You discover that you are actually taking the examination all the time: you are preparing for the examination by "taking" an examination, not by reading extraneous and/or supererogatory textbooks.

In short, this PASSBOOK®, used directedly, should be an important factor in helping you to pass your test.

CERTIFIED NURSE EXAMINATION SERIES

NURSING EXAMINATION RESOURCES

A variety of tests and programs are available through a number of organizations that will aid and help prepare candidates for nursing certification:

AMERICAN NURSES CREDENTIALING CENTER (ANCC)

The American Nurses Credentialing Center (ANCC) is a subsidiary of the American Nurses' Association (ANA), and the largest nursing credentialing organization in the United States. The ANCC Commission on Certification offers approximately 40 examinations including advanced practice specialties for nurse practitioners and clinical nurse specialists.

Certification is a most important way for you to show that you are among the best in your field – an extra step for you and your career, a step *beyond* state licensing. It gives you recognition and status on a *national* basis.

ANCC certification exams are offered twice a year in May and October in paper-and-pencil format, and throughout the year as computer-based exams. All exams are multiple choice and cover knowledge, understanding and application of professional nursing practice and theory. The time allotted for both the paper-and-pencil and computer certification exams is 3 hours and 30 minutes.

Each exam is developed in cooperation with an individual Content Expert Panel (CEP) composed of experts representing specific areas of certification. These panels analyze the professional skills and abilities required and then define which content should be covered and how strongly emphasized. Test questions are written by certified nurses in their discipline and reviewed by the ANCC to ensure validity and quality.

Exams are scored on a scale, and will be reported as either "Pass" or "Fail." Those who fail the exam will receive diagnostic information for each area of the test. There is a minimum 90-day waiting period from the date of the failed exam for those looking to retake it. For those who pass the exam, a certificate, official identification card and pin will be sent. Certification is valid for five years.

For further information and application for admission to candidacy for certification, write to:
American Nurses Credentialing Center
8515 Georgia Ave., Suite 400
Silver Spring, MD 20910-3492

You can also contact the ANCC and receive further details regarding certification exams and registration by visiting its home on the Internet – www.nursecredentialing.org – or by phone (1-800-284-CERT). Test Content Outlines (TCO) for each exam can also be found on the ANCC website, detailing the format and content breakdown of the test as well as the content areas the examinee should be prepared for.

NATIONAL CERTIFICATION CORPORATION

NCC CERTIFICATION

NCC – the National Certification Corporation for the Obstetric, Gynecologic and Neonatal Nursing specialties – is an independent certification organization. NCC was established in 1975 as a non-profit corporation for the purpose of sponsoring a volunteer certification program.

BENEFITS OF CERTIFICATION

Certification serves as an added credential to attest to attainment of special knowledge beyond the basic nursing degree. Certification serves to maintain and promote quality nursing care by providing a mechanism to nurses to demonstrate their special knowledge in a specific nursing area.

Promotion of quality care through certification benefits not only the individual nurse and the profession of nursing, but the public as well. Certification documents to employers, professional colleagues and health team members that special knowledge has been achieved, provides for expanded career opportunities and advancement within the specialty of OGN nursing, and elevates the standards of the obstetric, gynecologic and neonatal nursing practice.

Certification granted by NCC is pursuant to a voluntary procedure intended solely to test for special knowledge.

NCC does not purport to license, to confer a right or privilege upon, nor otherwise to define qualifications of any person for nursing practice.

The significance of certification in any jurisdiction or institution is the responsibility of the candidate to determine. The candidate should contact the appropriate state board of nursing or institution.

EXAMINATION DEVELOPMENT

NCC selects educators and practitioners in both nursing and medicine who possess expertise in the specialty areas within the obstetric, gynecologic and neonatal nursing and related fields to serve on the test committees. Responsibilities of the test committees include coordination of overall development of certification examinations and development of materials to assist candidates to assess readiness to participate in the certification process.

EXAMINATION DESCRIPTION

Each of the examinations consists of 200 multiple-choice questions. Two forms of each examination are often given to provide the opportunity to perform statistical procedures which ensure added reliability to the total examination process. The examinations are offered only in English and are designed to test special knowledge.

The examinations are given once each in the morning and afternoon, Monday through Friday, at more than 100 test centers. Four hours are allotted for completion of the examination.

THE CERTIFICATION PROCESS

1. Applicants must complete and file a certification application and appropriate documentation and fees
2. An acknowledgment postcard is sent to each applicant when NCC receives the application
3. Eligibility to participate is determined
4. Applicant is notified of eligibility status and eligible candidate receives a Candidate Guide to NCC Certification (4 to 6 weeks from receipt of application)
5. Candidates will schedule their own appointment for an examination time and location, and must take the exam within a 90-day period from notification of eligibility
6. Test administration occurs
7. Examinations are scored and analyzed
8. Candidates receive score reports upon completion of computerized testing (not paper testing)
9. Candidates are notified of certification status, receive information about certification maintenance and are later issued formal certificates

REVIEW COURSES AND NCC

NCC does not sponsor or endorse any review courses or materials for the certification examinations, because to do so would be a conflict of interest.

NCC is not affiliated with and does not provide input or information for any review courses or materials that other organizations may offer.

NCC views certification as an evaluative process. Eligibility criteria have been established to identify a minimum level of preparation for the exams.

CANDIDATE GUIDE TO NCC CERTIFICATION

Each candidate determined eligible to participate in the NCC certification process will be sent a Guide to NCC Certification. These guides can also be found online at the NCC website (www.nccnet.org). The Candidate Guides contain:

- General policies and procedures about the certification process
- Competency Statements that serve as a role description for the specialty nurse
- Expanded examination content outline
- Bibliography of references
- Sample questions to familiarize candidates with examination format (*These questions are not representative of exam content or difficulty level)

The Candidate Guide is not provided as study material, but to assist candidates in evaluating their own nursing practice as they prepare for the certification examination through identification of potential areas of strength and weakness.

SCORING OF EXAMINATIONS

Passing scores are determined based on a criterion-referenced system. Criterion passing scores are established by the NCC Board of Directors in conjunction with the NCC Test Committees using standard psychometric procedures.

Each question is statistically analyzed and evaluated with psychometric consultation, and scores are computed based on this evaluation.

Candidates who take the computerized form of the certification exam will receive their score reports upon completion of the exam. Those who take the paper/pencil exam will not receive their score reports for several weeks after administration.

NOTIFICATION AND AWARDING OF CERTIFICATION

Each candidate is notified of the success or failure to achieve certification. Successful candidates receive a formal certificate and will be able to use the initial RNC (Registered Nurse Certified) to indicate certification status.

Certification is awarded for a period of three years. Initial certification is effective from the date of notification to December 31 of the third full calendar year following notification. Subsequent periods of certification are subject to policies of the Certification Maintenance Program.

CERTIFICATION MAINTENANCE

The NCC Certification Maintenance Program allows the certified nurse to maintain NCC certification status.

Certification status must be maintained on an ongoing basis every three years through demonstration of approved continuing education or reexamination. Certification that is not maintained through the Certification Maintenance Program may only be regained by reexamination.

Specific information about the Certification Maintenance Program is provided to successful certification candidates and may also be obtained by contacting the NCC website (www.nccnet.org).

GENERAL POLICIES

All required practice experience/employment must have occurred while the applicant is/was a U.S. or Canadian RN. Graduate Nurse or Interim Permit status is acceptable, but must be indicated separately on the application form in addition to original licensure information.

NCC defines employment as practice in any of the following settings: direct patient care, educational institutions, administration or research.

When meeting educational requirements, all coursework, including that not directly related to specialty areas, thesis work and/or other program requirements must be completed at the time the application is filed.

It is the policy of NCC that no individual shall be excluded from the opportunity to participate in the NCC certification program on the basis of race, national origin, religion, sex, age or handicap.

All applications received are subject to the nonrefundable application fee ($250 paper/pencil; $300 computer).

Incomplete applications or applications submitted without appropriate fees will be returned and subject to all policies, fees and deadlines.

Applicants determined eligible (whether the candidate has been notified or not) and withdrawn will be subject to stated refund policies.

All NCC policies and requirements are subject to change without notice.

RETEST POLICIES

The NCC does not limit the number of times a candidate may retake the NCC Certification Examinations. Unsuccessful candidates who wish to be retested must reapply, submit all applicable fees and documentation, and re-establish eligibility.

Eligibility: All eligibility criteria of practice experience and/or educational preparation must be met by the time of application. It is the candidate's decision to choose the appropriate examination, based on the content outline, the individual's practice experience and NCC eligibility criteria.

Forms: All required forms must be submitted, and must include all requested information. If the forms are missing information, your application will be returned or you may be found ineligible to sit for the exam. Be sure the RN licensure information is completed. Be sure your documentation is signed by your supervisor or program director, with his/her title indicated, and the date the form is signed. Review your forms before you submit them.

Fees and Refunds: The proper fee must be submitted with your application or it will be returned.

For a current exam catalog containing current fees, terms, filing deadlines and exam dates, contact the NCC at www.nccnet.org, call (312) 951-0207 or fax at (312) 951-9475.

National Certification Corporation
PO Box 11082
Chicago, IL 60611-0082

CENTER FOR CERTIFICATION PREPARATION AND REVIEW

The Center for Certification Preparation and Review (CCPR) provides practice examinations developed by nurses and is intended to familiarize candidates with the content and feel of the real test. The CCPR practice examination identifies content areas of strength and weakness, provides examples of the type and format of questions that will appear on the examination, as well as information on how to focus additional study efforts.

The CCPR program consists of: study strategies, competency statements, content outline, 160-item examination, answer key and sample answer sheet, performance assessment grid, rationales for answers and cited references. Exams are available for inpatient obstetric, maternal newborn, neonatal intensive care and low-risk neonatal nursing, as well as neonatal nurse practitioner and women's health care nurse practitioner.

More information on ordering these practice exams can be found at www.ccprnet.org.

The National Certification Corporation (NCC), a not-for-profit organization that provides a national credentialing program for nurses, physicians and other licensed health care personnel, offers candidate guides for each of the NCC examinations. These candidate guides contain competency statements, detailed test outlines, sample questions, list of book/periodical references and all NCC policies related to the test administration process.

NCC guides are available in the following areas: inpatient obstetric, low-risk neonatal, maternal newborn and neonatal intensive care nursing, as well as neonatal nurse practitioner, telephone nursing practice, women's health care nurse practitioner, electronic fetal monitoring subspecialty examination, and menopause clinician. These guides, in addition to other information regarding testing, NCC publications and links to other organizations, are available online at www.nccnet.org.

RESOURCES FOR PRE-ADMISSION AND ACHIEVEMENT TESTS IN RN AND PN PROGRAMS

The National League for Nursing (NLN) offers a wide variety of examinations designed to aid students looking to further their education in the field of nursing. NLN pre-admission exams are reliable and valid predictors of student success in nursing programs, and NLN achievement tests allow educators to evaluate course or program objectives and to compare student performance to a national sample. The NLN also provides Diagnostic Readiness Tests, Critical Thinking and Comprehensive Nursing Achievement Exams and Acceleration Challenge Exams.

NLN exams can be ordered in paper form or e-mailed directly to you as online tests. The RN program includes tests in: basic nursing care, nursing care of children, maternity and child health nursing, nursing care of adults, psychiatric mental health and pharmacology in clinical nursing, baccalaureate achievement, physical assessment, community health nursing, comprehensive psychiatric nursing, heath and illness, anatomy and physiology, and microbiology.

NLN achievement tests also cover a PN program, which includes exams in: PN fundamentals, maternity infant, child health and adult health nursing, as well as mental health concepts and PN pharmacology.

NLN Pre-NCLEX Readiness Tests serve as practice and review for the NCLEX. Comprehensive Nursing Achievement, Critical Thinking and Diagnostic Readiness Tests are complementary to one another and help students prepare for nursing practice and to pass the NCLEX.

For in-depth information about the types of tests available, ordering, and additional NLN publications, including the NLN test catalog (available for download), visit www.nln.org.

HOW TO TAKE A TEST

I. YOU MUST PASS AN EXAMINATION

A. WHAT EVERY CANDIDATE SHOULD KNOW

Examination applicants often ask us for help in preparing for the written test. What can I study in advance? What kinds of questions will be asked? How will the test be given? How will the papers be graded?

As an applicant for a civil service examination, you may be wondering about some of these things. Our purpose here is to suggest effective methods of advance study and to describe civil service examinations.

Your chances for success on this examination can be increased if you know how to prepare. Those "pre-examination jitters" can be reduced if you know what to expect. You can even experience an adventure in good citizenship if you know why civil service exams are given.

B. WHY ARE CIVIL SERVICE EXAMINATIONS GIVEN?

Civil service examinations are important to you in two ways. As a citizen, you want public jobs filled by employees who know how to do their work. As a job seeker, you want a fair chance to compete for that job on an equal footing with other candidates. The best-known means of accomplishing this two-fold goal is the competitive examination.

Exams are widely publicized throughout the nation. They may be administered for jobs in federal, state, city, municipal, town or village governments or agencies.

Any citizen may apply, with some limitations, such as the age or residence of applicants. Your experience and education may be reviewed to see whether you meet the requirements for the particular examination. When these requirements exist, they are reasonable and applied consistently to all applicants. Thus, a competitive examination may cause you some uneasiness now, but it is your privilege and safeguard.

C. HOW ARE CIVIL SERVICE EXAMS DEVELOPED?

Examinations are carefully written by trained technicians who are specialists in the field known as "psychological measurement," in consultation with recognized authorities in the field of work that the test will cover. These experts recommend the subject matter areas or skills to be tested; only those knowledges or skills important to your success on the job are included. The most reliable books and source materials available are used as references. Together, the experts and technicians judge the difficulty level of the questions.

Test technicians know how to phrase questions so that the problem is clearly stated. Their ethics do not permit "trick" or "catch" questions. Questions may have been tried out on sample groups, or subjected to statistical analysis, to determine their usefulness.

Written tests are often used in combination with performance tests, ratings of training and experience, and oral interviews. All of these measures combine to form the best-known means of finding the right person for the right job.

II. HOW TO PASS THE WRITTEN TEST

A. NATURE OF THE EXAMINATION

To prepare intelligently for civil service examinations, you should know how they differ from school examinations you have taken. In school you were assigned certain definite pages to read or subjects to cover. The examination questions were quite detailed and usually emphasized memory. Civil service exams, on the other hand, try to discover your present ability to perform the duties of a position, plus your potentiality to learn these duties. In other words, a civil service exam attempts to predict how successful you will be. Questions cover such a broad area that they cannot be as minute and detailed as school exam questions.

In the public service similar kinds of work, or positions, are grouped together in one "class." This process is known as *position-classification*. All the positions in a class are paid according to the salary range for that class. One class title covers all of these positions, and they are all tested by the same examination.

B. FOUR BASIC STEPS

1) Study the announcement

How, then, can you know what subjects to study? Our best answer is: "Learn as much as possible about the class of positions for which you've applied." The exam will test the knowledge, skills and abilities needed to do the work.

Your most valuable source of information about the position you want is the official exam announcement. This announcement lists the training and experience qualifications. Check these standards and apply only if you come reasonably close to meeting them.

The brief description of the position in the examination announcement offers some clues to the subjects which will be tested. Think about the job itself. Review the duties in your mind. Can you perform them, or are there some in which you are rusty? Fill in the blank spots in your preparation.

Many jurisdictions preview the written test in the exam announcement by including a section called "Knowledge and Abilities Required," "Scope of the Examination," or some similar heading. Here you will find out specifically what fields will be tested.

2) Review your own background

Once you learn in general what the position is all about, and what you need to know to do the work, ask yourself which subjects you already know fairly well and which need improvement. You may wonder whether to concentrate on improving your strong areas or on building some background in your fields of weakness. When the announcement has specified "some knowledge" or "considerable knowledge," or has used adjectives like "beginning principles of..." or "advanced ... methods," you can get a clue as to the number and difficulty of questions to be asked in any given field. More questions, and hence broader coverage, would be included for those subjects which are more important in the work. Now weigh your strengths and weaknesses against the job requirements and prepare accordingly.

3) Determine the level of the position

Another way to tell how intensively you should prepare is to understand the level of the job for which you are applying. Is it the entering level? In other words, is this the position in which beginners in a field of work are hired? Or is it an intermediate or advanced level? Sometimes this is indicated by such words as "Junior" or "Senior" in the class title. Other jurisdictions use Roman numerals to designate the level – Clerk I, Clerk II, for example. The word "Supervisor" sometimes appears in the title. If the level is not indicated by the title, check the description of duties. Will you be working under very close supervision, or will you have responsibility for independent decisions in this work?

4) Choose appropriate study materials

Now that you know the subjects to be examined and the relative amount of each subject to be covered, you can choose suitable study materials. For beginning level jobs, or even advanced ones, if you have a pronounced weakness in some aspect of your training, read a modern, standard textbook in that field. Be sure it is up to date and has general coverage. Such books are normally available at your library, and the librarian will be glad to help you locate one. For entry-level positions, questions of appropriate difficulty are chosen – neither highly advanced questions, nor those too simple. Such questions require careful thought but not advanced training.

If the position for which you are applying is technical or advanced, you will read more advanced, specialized material. If you are already familiar with the basic principles of your field, elementary textbooks would waste your time. Concentrate on advanced textbooks and technical periodicals. Think through the concepts and review difficult problems in your field.

These are all general sources. You can get more ideas on your own initiative, following these leads. For example, training manuals and publications of the government agency which employs workers in your field can be useful, particularly for technical and professional positions. A letter or visit to the government department involved may result in more specific study suggestions, and certainly will provide you with a more definite idea of the exact nature of the position you are seeking.

III. KINDS OF TESTS

Tests are used for purposes other than measuring knowledge and ability to perform specified duties. For some positions, it is equally important to test ability to make adjustments to new situations or to profit from training. In others, basic mental abilities not dependent on information are essential. Questions which test these things may not appear as pertinent to the duties of the position as those which test for knowledge and information. Yet they are often highly important parts of a fair examination. For very general questions, it is almost impossible to help you direct your study efforts. What we can do is to point out some of the more common of these general abilities needed in public service positions and describe some typical questions.

1) General information

Broad, general information has been found useful for predicting job success in some kinds of work. This is tested in a variety of ways, from vocabulary lists to questions about current events. Basic background in some field of work, such as sociology or economics, may be sampled in a group of questions. Often these are principles which have become familiar to most persons through exposure rather than through formal training. It is difficult to advise you how to study for these questions; being alert to the world around you is our best suggestion.

2) Verbal ability

An example of an ability needed in many positions is verbal or language ability. Verbal ability is, in brief, the ability to use and understand words. Vocabulary and grammar tests are typical measures of this ability. Reading comprehension or paragraph interpretation questions are common in many kinds of civil service tests. You are given a paragraph of written material and asked to find its central meaning.

3) Numerical ability

Number skills can be tested by the familiar arithmetic problem, by checking paired lists of numbers to see which are alike and which are different, or by interpreting charts and graphs. In the latter test, a graph may be printed in the test booklet which you are asked to use as the basis for answering questions.

4) Observation

A popular test for law-enforcement positions is the observation test. A picture is shown to you for several minutes, then taken away. Questions about the picture test your ability to observe both details and larger elements.

5) Following directions

In many positions in the public service, the employee must be able to carry out written instructions dependably and accurately. You may be given a chart with several columns, each column listing a variety of information. The questions require you to carry out directions involving the information given in the chart.

6) Skills and aptitudes

Performance tests effectively measure some manual skills and aptitudes. When the skill is one in which you are trained, such as typing or shorthand, you can practice. These tests are often very much like those given in business school or high school courses. For many of the other skills and aptitudes, however, no short-time preparation can be made. Skills and abilities natural to you or that you have developed throughout your lifetime are being tested.

Many of the general questions just described provide all the data needed to answer the questions and ask you to use your reasoning ability to find the answers. Your best preparation for these tests, as well as for tests of facts and ideas, is to be at your physical and mental best. You, no doubt, have your own methods of getting into an exam-taking mood and keeping "in shape." The next section lists some ideas on this subject.

IV. KINDS OF QUESTIONS

Only rarely is the "essay" question, which you answer in narrative form, used in civil service tests. Civil service tests are usually of the short-answer type. Full instructions for answering these questions will be given to you at the examination. But in case this is your first experience with short-answer questions and separate answer sheets, here is what you need to know:

1) Multiple-choice Questions

Most popular of the short-answer questions is the "multiple choice" or "best answer" question. It can be used, for example, to test for factual knowledge, ability to solve problems or judgment in meeting situations found at work.

A multiple-choice question is normally one of three types—
- It can begin with an incomplete statement followed by several possible endings. You are to find the one ending which *best* completes the statement, although some of the others may not be entirely wrong.
- It can also be a complete statement in the form of a question which is answered by choosing one of the statements listed.

- It can be in the form of a problem – again you select the best answer.

Here is an example of a multiple-choice question with a discussion which should give you some clues as to the method for choosing the right answer:

When an employee has a complaint about his assignment, the action which will *best* help him overcome his difficulty is to
   A. discuss his difficulty with his coworkers
   B. take the problem to the head of the organization
   C. take the problem to the person who gave him the assignment
   D. say nothing to anyone about his complaint

In answering this question, you should study each of the choices to find which is best. Consider choice "A" – Certainly an employee may discuss his complaint with fellow employees, but no change or improvement can result, and the complaint remains unresolved. Choice "B" is a poor choice since the head of the organization probably does not know what assignment you have been given, and taking your problem to him is known as "going over the head" of the supervisor. The supervisor, or person who made the assignment, is the person who can clarify it or correct any injustice. Choice "C" is, therefore, correct. To say nothing, as in choice "D," is unwise. Supervisors have and interest in knowing the problems employees are facing, and the employee is seeking a solution to his problem.

2) True/False Questions

The "true/false" or "right/wrong" form of question is sometimes used. Here a complete statement is given. Your job is to decide whether the statement is right or wrong.

SAMPLE: A roaming cell-phone call to a nearby city costs less than a non-roaming call to a distant city.

This statement is wrong, or false, since roaming calls are more expensive.

This is not a complete list of all possible question forms, although most of the others are variations of these common types. You will always get complete directions for answering questions. Be sure you understand *how* to mark your answers – ask questions until you do.

V. RECORDING YOUR ANSWERS

Computer terminals are used more and more today for many different kinds of exams.

For an examination with very few applicants, you may be told to record your answers in the test booklet itself. Separate answer sheets are much more common. If this separate answer sheet is to be scored by machine – and this is often the case – it is highly important that you mark your answers correctly in order to get credit.

An electronic scoring machine is often used in civil service offices because of the speed with which papers can be scored. Machine-scored answer sheets must be marked with a pencil, which will be given to you. This pencil has a high graphite content which responds to the electronic scoring machine. As a matter of fact, stray dots may register as answers, so do not let your pencil rest on the answer sheet while you are pondering the correct answer. Also, if your pencil lead breaks or is otherwise defective, ask for another.

Since the answer sheet will be dropped in a slot in the scoring machine, be careful not to bend the corners or get the paper crumpled.

The answer sheet normally has five vertical columns of numbers, with 30 numbers to a column. These numbers correspond to the question numbers in your test booklet. After each number, going across the page are four or five pairs of dotted lines. These short dotted lines have small letters or numbers above them. The first two pairs may also have a "T" or "F" above the letters. This indicates that the first two pairs only are to be used if the questions are of the true-false type. If the questions are multiple choice, disregard the "T" and "F" and pay attention only to the small letters or numbers.

Answer your questions in the manner of the sample that follows:

32. The largest city in the United States is
   A. Washington, D.C.
   B. New York City
   C. Chicago
   D. Detroit
   E. San Francisco

1) Choose the answer you think is best. (New York City is the largest, so "B" is correct.)
2) Find the row of dotted lines numbered the same as the question you are answering. (Find row number 32)
3) Find the pair of dotted lines corresponding to the answer. (Find the pair of lines under the mark "B.")
4) Make a solid black mark between the dotted lines.

VI. BEFORE THE TEST

Common sense will help you find procedures to follow to get ready for an examination. Too many of us, however, overlook these sensible measures. Indeed, nervousness and fatigue have been found to be the most serious reasons why applicants fail to do their best on civil service tests. Here is a list of reminders:

- Begin your preparation early – Don't wait until the last minute to go scurrying around for books and materials or to find out what the position is all about.
- Prepare continuously – An hour a night for a week is better than an all-night cram session. This has been definitely established. What is more, a night a week for a month will return better dividends than crowding your study into a shorter period of time.
- Locate the place of the exam – You have been sent a notice telling you when and where to report for the examination. If the location is in a different town or otherwise unfamiliar to you, it would be well to inquire the best route and learn something about the building.
- Relax the night before the test – Allow your mind to rest. Do not study at all that night. Plan some mild recreation or diversion; then go to bed early and get a good night's sleep.
- Get up early enough to make a leisurely trip to the place for the test – This way unforeseen events, traffic snarls, unfamiliar buildings, etc. will not upset you.
- Dress comfortably – A written test is not a fashion show. You will be known by number and not by name, so wear something comfortable.

- Leave excess paraphernalia at home – Shopping bags and odd bundles will get in your way. You need bring only the items mentioned in the official notice you received; usually everything you need is provided. Do not bring reference books to the exam. They will only confuse those last minutes and be taken away from you when in the test room.
- Arrive somewhat ahead of time – If because of transportation schedules you must get there very early, bring a newspaper or magazine to take your mind off yourself while waiting.
- Locate the examination room – When you have found the proper room, you will be directed to the seat or part of the room where you will sit. Sometimes you are given a sheet of instructions to read while you are waiting. Do not fill out any forms until you are told to do so; just read them and be prepared.
- Relax and prepare to listen to the instructions
- If you have any physical problem that may keep you from doing your best, be sure to tell the test administrator. If you are sick or in poor health, you really cannot do your best on the exam. You can come back and take the test some other time.

VII. AT THE TEST

The day of the test is here and you have the test booklet in your hand. The temptation to get going is very strong. Caution! There is more to success than knowing the right answers. You must know how to identify your papers and understand variations in the type of short-answer question used in this particular examination. Follow these suggestions for maximum results from your efforts:

1) Cooperate with the monitor

The test administrator has a duty to create a situation in which you can be as much at ease as possible. He will give instructions, tell you when to begin, check to see that you are marking your answer sheet correctly, and so on. He is not there to guard you, although he will see that your competitors do not take unfair advantage. He wants to help you do your best.

2) Listen to all instructions

Don't jump the gun! Wait until you understand all directions. In most civil service tests you get more time than you need to answer the questions. So don't be in a hurry. Read each word of instructions until you clearly understand the meaning. Study the examples, listen to all announcements and follow directions. Ask questions if you do not understand what to do.

3) Identify your papers

Civil service exams are usually identified by number only. You will be assigned a number; you must not put your name on your test papers. Be sure to copy your number correctly. Since more than one exam may be given, copy your exact examination title.

4) Plan your time

Unless you are told that a test is a "speed" or "rate of work" test, speed itself is usually not important. Time enough to answer all the questions will be provided, but this does not mean that you have all day. An overall time limit has been set. Divide the total time (in minutes) by the number of questions to determine the approximate time you have for each question.

5) Do not linger over difficult questions

If you come across a difficult question, mark it with a paper clip (useful to have along) and come back to it when you have been through the booklet. One caution if you do this – be sure to skip a number on your answer sheet as well. Check often to be sure that you have not lost your place and that you are marking in the row numbered the same as the question you are answering.

6) Read the questions

Be sure you know what the question asks! Many capable people are unsuccessful because they failed to *read* the questions correctly.

7) Answer all questions

Unless you have been instructed that a penalty will be deducted for incorrect answers, it is better to guess than to omit a question.

8) Speed tests

It is often better NOT to guess on speed tests. It has been found that on timed tests people are tempted to spend the last few seconds before time is called in marking answers at random – without even reading them – in the hope of picking up a few extra points. To discourage this practice, the instructions may warn you that your score will be "corrected" for guessing. That is, a penalty will be applied. The incorrect answers will be deducted from the correct ones, or some other penalty formula will be used.

9) Review your answers

If you finish before time is called, go back to the questions you guessed or omitted to give them further thought. Review other answers if you have time.

10) Return your test materials

If you are ready to leave before others have finished or time is called, take ALL your materials to the monitor and leave quietly. Never take any test material with you. The monitor can discover whose papers are not complete, and taking a test booklet may be grounds for disqualification.

VIII. EXAMINATION TECHNIQUES

1) Read the general instructions carefully. These are usually printed on the first page of the exam booklet. As a rule, these instructions refer to the timing of the examination; the fact that you should not start work until the signal and must stop work at a signal, etc. If there are any *special* instructions, such as a choice of questions to be answered, make sure that you note this instruction carefully.

2) When you are ready to start work on the examination, that is as soon as the signal has been given, read the instructions to each question booklet, underline any key words or phrases, such as *least, best, outline, describe* and the like. In this way you will tend to answer as requested rather than discover on reviewing your paper that you *listed without describing*, that you selected the *worst* choice rather than the *best* choice, etc.

3) If the examination is of the objective or multiple-choice type – that is, each question will also give a series of possible answers: A, B, C or D, and you are called upon to select the best answer and write the letter next to that answer on your answer paper – it is advisable to start answering each question in turn. There may be anywhere from 50 to 100 such questions in the three or four hours allotted and you can see how much time would be taken if you read through all the questions before beginning to answer any. Furthermore, if you come across a question or group of questions which you know would be difficult to answer, it would undoubtedly affect your handling of all the other questions.

4) If the examination is of the essay type and contains but a few questions, it is a moot point as to whether you should read all the questions before starting to answer any one. Of course, if you are given a choice – say five out of seven and the like – then it is essential to read all the questions so you can eliminate the two that are most difficult. If, however, you are asked to answer all the questions, there may be danger in trying to answer the easiest one first because you may find that you will spend too much time on it. The best technique is to answer the first question, then proceed to the second, etc.

5) Time your answers. Before the exam begins, write down the time it started, then add the time allowed for the examination and write down the time it must be completed, then divide the time available somewhat as follows:
    - If 3-1/2 hours are allowed, that would be 210 minutes. If you have 80 objective-type questions, that would be an average of 2-1/2 minutes per question. Allow yourself no more than 2 minutes per question, or a total of 160 minutes, which will permit about 50 minutes to review.
    - If for the time allotment of 210 minutes there are 7 essay questions to answer, that would average about 30 minutes a question. Give yourself only 25 minutes per question so that you have about 35 minutes to review.

6) The most important instruction is to *read each question* and make sure you know what is wanted. The second most important instruction is to *time yourself properly* so that you answer every question. The third most important instruction is to *answer every question*. Guess if you have to but include something for each question. Remember that you will receive no credit for a blank and will probably receive some credit if you write something in answer to an essay question. If you guess a letter – say "B" for a multiple-choice question – you may have guessed right. If you leave a blank as an answer to a multiple-choice question, the examiners may respect your feelings but it will not add a point to your score. Some exams may penalize you for wrong answers, so in such cases *only*, you may not want to guess unless you have some basis for your answer.

7) Suggestions
    a. Objective-type questions
        1. Examine the question booklet for proper sequence of pages and questions
        2. Read all instructions carefully
        3. Skip any question which seems too difficult; return to it after all other questions have been answered
        4. Apportion your time properly; do not spend too much time on any single question or group of questions

5. Note and underline key words – *all, most, fewest, least, best, worst, same, opposite,* etc.
6. Pay particular attention to negatives
7. Note unusual option, e.g., unduly long, short, complex, different or similar in content to the body of the question
8. Observe the use of "hedging" words – *probably, may, most likely,* etc.
9. Make sure that your answer is put next to the same number as the question
10. Do not second-guess unless you have good reason to believe the second answer is definitely more correct
11. Cross out original answer if you decide another answer is more accurate; do not erase until you are ready to hand your paper in
12. Answer all questions; guess unless instructed otherwise
13. Leave time for review

b. Essay questions
1. Read each question carefully
2. Determine exactly what is wanted. Underline key words or phrases.
3. Decide on outline or paragraph answer
4. Include many different points and elements unless asked to develop any one or two points or elements
5. Show impartiality by giving pros and cons unless directed to select one side only
6. Make and write down any assumptions you find necessary to answer the questions
7. Watch your English, grammar, punctuation and choice of words
8. Time your answers; don't crowd material

8) Answering the essay question

Most essay questions can be answered by framing the specific response around several key words or ideas. Here are a few such key words or ideas:

M's: manpower, materials, methods, money, management
P's: purpose, program, policy, plan, procedure, practice, problems, pitfalls, personnel, public relations

a. Six basic steps in handling problems:
1. Preliminary plan and background development
2. Collect information, data and facts
3. Analyze and interpret information, data and facts
4. Analyze and develop solutions as well as make recommendations
5. Prepare report and sell recommendations
6. Install recommendations and follow up effectiveness

b. Pitfalls to avoid
1. *Taking things for granted* – A statement of the situation does not necessarily imply that each of the elements is necessarily true; for example, a complaint may be invalid and biased so that all that can be taken for granted is that a complaint has been registered

2. *Considering only one side of a situation* – Wherever possible, indicate several alternatives and then point out the reasons you selected the best one
3. *Failing to indicate follow up* – Whenever your answer indicates action on your part, make certain that you will take proper follow-up action to see how successful your recommendations, procedures or actions turn out to be
4. *Taking too long in answering any single question* – Remember to time your answers properly

IX. AFTER THE TEST

Scoring procedures differ in detail among civil service jurisdictions although the general principles are the same. Whether the papers are hand-scored or graded by machine we have described, they are nearly always graded by number. That is, the person who marks the paper knows only the number – never the name – of the applicant. Not until all the papers have been graded will they be matched with names. If other tests, such as training and experience or oral interview ratings have been given, scores will be combined. Different parts of the examination usually have different weights. For example, the written test might count 60 percent of the final grade, and a rating of training and experience 40 percent. In many jurisdictions, veterans will have a certain number of points added to their grades.

After the final grade has been determined, the names are placed in grade order and an eligible list is established. There are various methods for resolving ties between those who get the same final grade – probably the most common is to place first the name of the person whose application was received first. Job offers are made from the eligible list in the order the names appear on it. You will be notified of your grade and your rank as soon as all these computations have been made. This will be done as rapidly as possible.

People who are found to meet the requirements in the announcement are called "eligibles." Their names are put on a list of eligible candidates. An eligible's chances of getting a job depend on how high he stands on this list and how fast agencies are filling jobs from the list.

When a job is to be filled from a list of eligibles, the agency asks for the names of people on the list of eligibles for that job. When the civil service commission receives this request, it sends to the agency the names of the three people highest on this list. Or, if the job to be filled has specialized requirements, the office sends the agency the names of the top three persons who meet these requirements from the general list.

The appointing officer makes a choice from among the three people whose names were sent to him. If the selected person accepts the appointment, the names of the others are put back on the list to be considered for future openings.

That is the rule in hiring from all kinds of eligible lists, whether they are for typist, carpenter, chemist, or something else. For every vacancy, the appointing officer has his choice of any one of the top three eligibles on the list. This explains why the person whose name is on top of the list sometimes does not get an appointment when some of the persons lower on the list do. If the appointing officer chooses the second or third eligible, the No. 1 eligible does not get a job at once, but stays on the list until he is appointed or the list is terminated.

X. HOW TO PASS THE INTERVIEW TEST

The examination for which you applied requires an oral interview test. You have already taken the written test and you are now being called for the interview test – the final part of the formal examination.

You may think that it is not possible to prepare for an interview test and that there are no procedures to follow during an interview. Our purpose is to point out some things you can do in advance that will help you and some good rules to follow and pitfalls to avoid while you are being interviewed.

What is an interview supposed to test?

The written examination is designed to test the technical knowledge and competence of the candidate; the oral is designed to evaluate intangible qualities, not readily measured otherwise, and to establish a list showing the relative fitness of each candidate – as measured against his competitors – for the position sought. Scoring is not on the basis of "right" and "wrong," but on a sliding scale of values ranging from "not passable" to "outstanding." As a matter of fact, it is possible to achieve a relatively low score without a single "incorrect" answer because of evident weakness in the qualities being measured.

Occasionally, an examination may consist entirely of an oral test – either an individual or a group oral. In such cases, information is sought concerning the technical knowledges and abilities of the candidate, since there has been no written examination for this purpose. More commonly, however, an oral test is used to supplement a written examination.

Who conducts interviews?

The composition of oral boards varies among different jurisdictions. In nearly all, a representative of the personnel department serves as chairman. One of the members of the board may be a representative of the department in which the candidate would work. In some cases, "outside experts" are used, and, frequently, a businessman or some other representative of the general public is asked to serve. Labor and management or other special groups may be represented. The aim is to secure the services of experts in the appropriate field.

However the board is composed, it is a good idea (and not at all improper or unethical) to ascertain in advance of the interview who the members are and what groups they represent. When you are introduced to them, you will have some idea of their backgrounds and interests, and at least you will not stutter and stammer over their names.

What should be done before the interview?

While knowledge about the board members is useful and takes some of the surprise element out of the interview, there is other preparation which is more substantive. It *is* possible to prepare for an oral interview – in several ways:

1) Keep a copy of your application and review it carefully before the interview

This may be the only document before the oral board, and the starting point of the interview. Know what education and experience you have listed there, and the sequence and dates of all of it. Sometimes the board will ask you to review the highlights of your experience for them; you should not have to hem and haw doing it.

2) Study the class specification and the examination announcement

Usually, the oral board has one or both of these to guide them. The qualities, characteristics or knowledges required by the position sought are stated in these documents. They offer valuable clues as to the nature of the oral interview. For example, if the job involves supervisory responsibilities, the announcement will usually indicate that knowledge of modern supervisory methods and the qualifications of the candidate as a supervisor will be tested. If so, you can expect such questions, frequently in the form of a hypothetical situation which you are expected to solve. NEVER go into an oral without knowledge of the duties and responsibilities of the job you seek.

3) Think through each qualification required

Try to visualize the kind of questions you would ask if you were a board member. How well could you answer them? Try especially to appraise your own knowledge and background in each area, *measured against the job sought*, and identify any areas in which you are weak. Be critical and realistic – do not flatter yourself.

4) Do some general reading in areas in which you feel you may be weak

For example, if the job involves supervision and your past experience has NOT, some general reading in supervisory methods and practices, particularly in the field of human relations, might be useful. Do NOT study agency procedures or detailed manuals. The oral board will be testing your understanding and capacity, not your memory.

5) Get a good night's sleep and watch your general health and mental attitude

You will want a clear head at the interview. Take care of a cold or any other minor ailment, and of course, no hangovers.

What should be done on the day of the interview?

Now comes the day of the interview itself. Give yourself plenty of time to get there. Plan to arrive somewhat ahead of the scheduled time, particularly if your appointment is in the fore part of the day. If a previous candidate fails to appear, the board might be ready for you a bit early. By early afternoon an oral board is almost invariably behind schedule if there are many candidates, and you may have to wait. Take along a book or magazine to read, or your application to review, but leave any extraneous material in the waiting room when you go in for your interview. In any event, relax and compose yourself.

The matter of dress is important. The board is forming impressions about you – from your experience, your manners, your attitude, and your appearance. Give your personal appearance careful attention. Dress your best, but not your flashiest. Choose conservative, appropriate clothing, and be sure it is immaculate. This is a business interview, and your appearance should indicate that you regard it as such. Besides, being well groomed and properly dressed will help boost your confidence.

Sooner or later, someone will call your name and escort you into the interview room. *This is it.* From here on you are on your own. It is too late for any more preparation. But remember, you asked for this opportunity to prove your fitness, and you are here because your request was granted.

What happens when you go in?

The usual sequence of events will be as follows: The clerk (who is often the board stenographer) will introduce you to the chairman of the oral board, who will introduce you to the other members of the board. Acknowledge the introductions before you sit down. Do not be surprised if you find a microphone facing you or a stenotypist sitting by. Oral interviews are usually recorded in the event of an appeal or other review.

Usually the chairman of the board will open the interview by reviewing the highlights of your education and work experience from your application – primarily for the benefit of the other members of the board, as well as to get the material into the record. Do not interrupt or comment unless there is an error or significant misinterpretation; if that is the case, do not hesitate. But do not quibble about insignificant matters. Also, he will usually ask you some question about your education, experience or your present job – partly to get you to start talking and to establish the interviewing "rapport." He may start the actual questioning, or turn it over to one of the other members. Frequently, each member undertakes the questioning on a particular area, one in which he is perhaps most competent, so you can expect each member to participate in the examination. Because time is limited, you may also expect some rather abrupt switches in the direction the questioning takes, so do not be upset by it. Normally, a board member will not pursue a single line of questioning unless he discovers a particular strength or weakness.

After each member has participated, the chairman will usually ask whether any member has any further questions, then will ask you if you have anything you wish to add. Unless you are expecting this question, it may floor you. Worse, it may start you off on an extended, extemporaneous speech. The board is not usually seeking more information. The question is principally to offer you a last opportunity to present further qualifications or to indicate that you have nothing to add. So, if you feel that a significant qualification or characteristic has been overlooked, it is proper to point it out in a sentence or so. Do not compliment the board on the thoroughness of their examination – they have been sketchy, and you know it. If you wish, merely say, "No thank you, I have nothing further to add." This is a point where you can "talk yourself out" of a good impression or fail to present an important bit of information. Remember, *you close the interview yourself.*

The chairman will then say, "That is all, Mr. _____, thank you." Do not be startled; the interview is over, and quicker than you think. Thank him, gather your belongings and take your leave. Save your sigh of relief for the other side of the door.

How to put your best foot forward

Throughout this entire process, you may feel that the board individually and collectively is trying to pierce your defenses, seek out your hidden weaknesses and embarrass and confuse you. Actually, this is not true. They are obliged to make an appraisal of your qualifications for the job you are seeking, and they want to see you in your best light. Remember, they must interview all candidates and a non-cooperative candidate may become a failure in spite of their best efforts to bring out his qualifications. Here are 15 suggestions that will help you:

1) Be natural – Keep your attitude confident, not cocky

If you are not confident that you can do the job, do not expect the board to be. Do not apologize for your weaknesses, try to bring out your strong points. The board is interested in a positive, not negative, presentation. Cockiness will antagonize any board member and make him wonder if you are covering up a weakness by a false show of strength.

2) Get comfortable, but don't lounge or sprawl

Sit erectly but not stiffly. A careless posture may lead the board to conclude that you are careless in other things, or at least that you are not impressed by the importance of the occasion. Either conclusion is natural, even if incorrect. Do not fuss with your clothing, a pencil or an ashtray. Your hands may occasionally be useful to emphasize a point; do not let them become a point of distraction.

3) Do not wisecrack or make small talk

This is a serious situation, and your attitude should show that you consider it as such. Further, the time of the board is limited – they do not want to waste it, and neither should you.

4) Do not exaggerate your experience or abilities

In the first place, from information in the application or other interviews and sources, the board may know more about you than you think. Secondly, you probably will not get away with it. An experienced board is rather adept at spotting such a situation, so do not take the chance.

5) If you know a board member, do not make a point of it, yet do not hide it

Certainly you are not fooling him, and probably not the other members of the board. Do not try to take advantage of your acquaintanceship – it will probably do you little good.

6) Do not dominate the interview

Let the board do that. They will give you the clues – do not assume that you have to do all the talking. Realize that the board has a number of questions to ask you, and do not try to take up all the interview time by showing off your extensive knowledge of the answer to the first one.

7) Be attentive

You only have 20 minutes or so, and you should keep your attention at its sharpest throughout. When a member is addressing a problem or question to you, give him your undivided attention. Address your reply principally to him, but do not exclude the other board members.

8) Do not interrupt

A board member may be stating a problem for you to analyze. He will ask you a question when the time comes. Let him state the problem, and wait for the question.

9) Make sure you understand the question

Do not try to answer until you are sure what the question is. If it is not clear, restate it in your own words or ask the board member to clarify it for you. However, do not haggle about minor elements.

10) Reply promptly but not hastily

A common entry on oral board rating sheets is "candidate responded readily," or "candidate hesitated in replies." Respond as promptly and quickly as you can, but do not jump to a hasty, ill-considered answer.

11) Do not be peremptory in your answers

A brief answer is proper – but do not fire your answer back. That is a losing game from your point of view. The board member can probably ask questions much faster than you can answer them.

12) Do not try to create the answer you think the board member wants

He is interested in what kind of mind you have and how it works – not in playing games. Furthermore, he can usually spot this practice and will actually grade you down on it.

13) Do not switch sides in your reply merely to agree with a board member

Frequently, a member will take a contrary position merely to draw you out and to see if you are willing and able to defend your point of view. Do not start a debate, yet do not surrender a good position. If a position is worth taking, it is worth defending.

14) Do not be afraid to admit an error in judgment if you are shown to be wrong

The board knows that you are forced to reply without any opportunity for careful consideration. Your answer may be demonstrably wrong. If so, admit it and get on with the interview.

15) Do not dwell at length on your present job

The opening question may relate to your present assignment. Answer the question but do not go into an extended discussion. You are being examined for a *new* job, not your present one. As a matter of fact, try to phrase ALL your answers in terms of the job for which you are being examined.

Basis of Rating

Probably you will forget most of these "do's" and "don'ts" when you walk into the oral interview room. Even remembering them all will not ensure you a passing grade. Perhaps you did not have the qualifications in the first place. But remembering them will help you to put your best foot forward, without treading on the toes of the board members.

Rumor and popular opinion to the contrary notwithstanding, an oral board wants you to make the best appearance possible. They know you are under pressure – but they also want to see how you respond to it as a guide to what your reaction would be under the pressures of the job you seek. They will be influenced by the degree of poise you display, the personal traits you show and the manner in which you respond.

ABOUT THIS BOOK

This book contains tests divided into Examination Sections. Go through each test, answering every question in the margin. We have also attached a sample answer sheet at the back of the book that can be removed and used. At the end of each test look at the answer key and check your answers. On the ones you got wrong, look at the right answer choice and learn. Do not fill in the answers first. Do not memorize the questions and answers, but understand the answer and principles involved. On your test, the questions will likely be different from the samples. Questions are changed and new ones added. If you understand these past questions you should have success with any changes that arise. Tests may consist of several types of questions. We have additional books on each subject should more study be advisable or necessary for you. Finally, the more you study, the better prepared you will be. This book is intended to be the last thing you study before you walk into the examination room. Prior study of relevant texts is also recommended. NLC publishes some of these in our Fundamental Series. Knowledge and good sense are important factors in passing your exam. Good luck also helps. So now study this Passbook, absorb the material contained within and take that knowledge into the examination. Then do your best to pass that exam.

EXAMINATION SECTION

EXAMINATION SECTION
TEST 1

DIRECTIONS: Each question or incomplete statement is followed by several suggested answers or completions. Select the one that BEST answers the question or completes the statement. *PRINT THE LETTER OF THE CORRECT ANSWER IN THE SPACE AT THE RIGHT.*

1. Normal inspiration is an active process that uses the diaphragm and external intercostal muscles.
   Ineffective breathing patterns can be manifested by all of the following EXCEPT

   A. use of accessory muscles for respiration
   B. increased breath sounds in lung segments
   C. paradoxical respiratory movement
   D. restlessness, anxiety, and diaphoresis

   1.____

2. Postural drainage is indicated for patients who have difficulty clearing secretions due to airway obstruction and/or excessive mucus production.
   Signs of airway obstruction include

   A. tachycardia
   B. increased breath sounds with no crackles or gurgles
   C. increased oxygen saturation
   D. decreased respiratory rate

   2.____

3. Therapeutic percussion is typically provided while the patient is in various PD positions.
   Percussions and vibrations are CONTRAINDICATED in

   A. spinal anesthesia B. thoracic skin grafts
   C. subcutaneous emphysema D. all of the above

   3.____

4. It may be inappropriate to simply administer oxygen without conducting a thorough patient assessment to determine the cause of the hypoxemic event.
   Oxygen therapy is commonly prescribed in the initial treatment of all of the following conditions EXCEPT

   A. acute myocardial infarction
   B. tuberculosis
   C. severe trauma
   D. immediately following surgery or extubation

   4.____

5. Breathing oxygen concentrations greater than 50% for more than 24 hours can cause injury to the lung tissue or oxygen toxicity.
   Early signs of oxygen toxicity include
      I. dyspnea, cough, lethargy, and vomiting
      II. restlessness
      III. retrosternal chest pain
      IV. hemoptasis
   The CORRECT answer is:

   A. I, II, III B. I, II, IV
   C. I, III, IV D. II, IV

   5.____

6. Some patients continue oxygen therapy following discharge. Indications for home oxygen therapy include all of the following EXCEPT

    A. pulmonary hypertension
    B. recurring congestive heart failure
    C. anemia
    D. sleep apnea syndrome

7. Oxygen will not explode, but will cause something on fire to burn much faster. Important precautionary measures to prevent fire include

    A. no smoking in any room where oxygen is being used
    B. keep equipment at least 10 feet away from any open flame
    C. do not use oily lotions, face creams, grease, or lip balms around oxygen equipment
    D. all of the above

8. A transtracheal oxygen catheter is a thin, teflon-coated tube that is surgically placed into the trachea.
Complications of transtracheal oxygen therapy include all of the following EXCEPT

    A. inflammation   B. thin secretions
    C. bleeding   D. infection

9. A metered-dose inhaler is a pressurized canister which releases an aerosol containing the drug suspended in a fluorocarbon gas stream.
The nurse should provide the patient with instructions to

    A. assemble the inhaler
    B. shake the inhaler to mix the medication and propellant
    C. remove the cap from the mouthpiece
    D. all of the above

10. Artificial airways are devices designed to maintain patent communication between the tracheobronchial tree and the air supply in the external environment.
Indications for an endotracheal tube include all of the following EXCEPT

    A. temporary measures for airway obstruction
    B. mechanical ventilation
    C. protection of nasal mucosa
    D. management of secretions

11. The main indication for the insertion of a nasal airway is to protect the nasal mucosa from the trauma of frequent passage of suction catheters.
A MAJOR disadvantage of nasal airway insertion is

    A. it does not prevent occlusion of upper airway by tongue
    B. potential inability to speak
    C. potential for aspiration
    D. potential for laryngeal damage

12. For long-term use, tracheostomy is preferred over endotracheal intubation. Advantages of tracheostomy tubes include all of the following EXCEPT

    A. direct communication with trachea
    B. longer tube length results in less airway resistance than with endotracheal tubes
    C. easily tolerated by patients
    D. avoidance of trauma to larynx

13. Complications of intubation can be mechanical or physiologic in nature. _____ is a physiologic, not a mechanical, complication.

    A. Tube displacement
    B. Obstruction
    C. Aspiration
    D. Loss of cuff seal

14. Nursing diagnoses for patients on mechanical ventilation include nursing diagnoses common to intubated patients, such as

    A. inadequate gas exchange related to increased secretions, interstitial edema, and shunt
    B. high risk for decreased cardiac output related to decreased venous return
    C. anxiety related to mechanical ventilation and severity of illness
    D. all of the above

15. Acute sinusitis commonly accompanies or follows an upper respiratory tract infection. Of the following, the LEAST commonly involved organism is

    A. C. defficle
    B. H. influenzae
    C. S. pyogens
    D. S. pneumoniae

16. Anaerobic pathogens are the most common infectious cause of chronic sinusitis. Non-infectious contributors to chronic sinusitis include all of the following EXCEPT

    A. smoking
    B. amphetamine abuse
    C. habitual nasal sprays or inhalants
    D. history of allergy

17. Rhinitis is commonly caused by viral infection, as in acute rhinitis, or the common cold, coryza.
    Known organisms in acute viral rhinitis include
    I. rhinovirus
    II. influenza and para-influenza
    III. infectious mononucleosis
    IV. coxsackie virus
    The CORRECT answer is:

    A. I, II, III
    B. II, III
    C. I, II, IV
    D. I, II, III, IV

18. Nursing interventions to educate patients with rhinitis in order to prevent further infection include all of the following EXCEPT

    A. disposing of tissues properly
    B. using cloth handkerchiefs
    C. using good handwashing techniques
    D. covering mouth and nose when coughing and sneezing

19. Nasal obstruction is commonly caused by displacement of the nasal septum from the midline position.
Common results of nasal deviation include

    A. nasal obstruction
    B. postnasal drip
    C. epistaxis
    D. all of the above

20. The priority of goals established for the patient with epistaxis will depend on the severity of the problem and the presence or absence of associated complications. APPROPRIATE goals for patients with epistaxis include

    A. normal vital signs and level of consciousness
    B. adequate caloric intake
    C. pain relief
    D. all of the above

21. Nursing interventions while taking care of a patient with epistaxis include all of the following EXCEPT

    A. immediate assessment of vital signs
    B. positioning of the patient with foot end of the bed elevated
    C. pressure applied to the nose
    D. coaching in mouth breathing

22. When evaluating the care of a patient with epistaxis, the nurse considers which of the following assessment parameters?
    I. Respiratory accessory muscles should not be used.
    II. Cyanosis and diaphoresis should be absent.
    III. Mucus membrane should remain pink and moist.
The CORRECT answer is:

    A. I only
    B. I, II
    C. I, II, III
    D. II, III

23. The priority of goals established for the patient with a nasal fracture will depend on the severity of the problem and the presence or absence of associated complications. Appropriate goals for a patient with this problem include all of the following EXCEPT

    A. patent airway and normal blood gas levels
    B. elevated body temperature
    C. pain relief
    D. verbalization of acceptance of temporary disfigurement

24. The most common form of laryngeal cancer is squamous cell carcinoma.
The one of the following which is NOT a risk factor for laryngeal squamous cell carcinoma is

    A. cocaine abuse
    B. prolonged use of tobacco and alcohol
    C. exposure to radiation
    D. voice abuse

25. The earliest symptom of laryngeal cancer is hoarseness, or voice change.
Later manifestations include all of the following EXCEPT

    A. increasing dyspnea
    B. hematemesis
    C. dysphagia
    D. hemoptysis

KEY (CORRECT ANSWERS)

1. B
2. A
3. D
4. B
5. A

6. C
7. D
8. B
9. D
10. C

11. A
12. B
13. C
14. D
15. A

16. B
17. C
18. B
19. D
20. D

21. B
22. C
23. B
24. A
25. B

TEST 2

DIRECTIONS: Each question or incomplete statement is followed by several suggested answers or completions. Select the one that BEST answers the question or completes the statement. *PRINT THE LETTER OF THE CORRECT ANSWER IN THE SPACE AT THE RIGHT.*

1. An important role of the nurse is to instruct and assist the patient in producing an effective cough.
Factors that influence the ability to cough include all of the following EXCEPT

    A. analgesia may be needed before cough exercise
    B. oral hydration using ice chips or sips of water can make coughing easier
    C. a lying down position is the most effective and comfortable position
    D. splinting a painful area during coughing with gentle hand pressure helps the patient cough

    1.____

2. Chronic obstructive pulmonary disease (COPD) is a broad term used to describe conditions characterized by chronic obstruction to expiratory air flow.
Complications of COPD include all of the following EXCEPT

    A. acute respiratory failure
    B. tuberculosis
    C. cor pulmonale
    D. pneumothorax

    2.____

3. The priority goals of nursing intervention for patients with acute exacerbation of COPD are the maintenance of adequate oxygenation, ventilation, and airway clearance. The patient should display

    A. clear breath sounds with no crackles
    B. respiratory rate between 12-20 breaths/minute at rest
    C. arterial PO_2 at patient's normal baseline
    D. all of the above

    3.____

4. The etiological factors of asthma are not completely understood, but it is clear that asthma can develop after exposure to a variety of substances.
Asthma is characterized by all of the following EXCEPT

    A. hemoptosis
    B. reversible airway obstruction
    C. airway inflammation
    D. airway hyperresponsiveness

    4.____

5. The severity of an asthma attack is reflected by the degree of airflow obstruction, level of oxygenation, and nature of breathing patterns.
Patients at increased risk for life-threatening asthma attacks do NOT include those

    A. less than 1 year old
    B. with PEFR or FEV_1 below 25% of predicted level
    C. with PCO_2 below 40 mmHg
    D. with wide daily fluctuation in PEFR or FEV_1

    5.____

6. Which of the following is associated with an acute asthma attack?
    I. Impaired gas exchange related to ventilation-per-fusion mismatch, impaired diffusion, or arterio-venous shunting
    II. Fatigue related to increased efforts to breathe
    III. Fluid volume deficit related to increased intake and decreased insensible loss

    The CORRECT answer is:

    A. I only
    B. I, II
    C. I, II, III
    D. II, III

7. Outcome criteria for a patient with asthma include all of the following EXCEPT that the patient

    A. maintain PaCO$_2$ at approximately 40 mmHg
    B. have clear breath sounds on auscultation
    C. maintain PaO$_2$ at approximately 50 mmHg
    D. report no breathlessness at rest and minimal with activities

8. Restrictive lung diseases encompass a vast array of disorders that lead to decreased lung inflation.
    A hallmark of all restrictive disorders, regardless of cause, is

    A. decreased lung volume
    B. decreased breath sounds
    C. decreased vital capacity
    D. increased residual volume

9. Restrictive disorders are associated with

    A. ineffective breathing pattern related to increased lung inflation
    B. impaired gas exchange related to increased surface area for diffusion
    C. activity intolerance related to impaired gas exchange
    D. all of the above

10. Adult respiratory distress syndrome (ARDS) is a common problem, and 65% of cases are fatal.
    Major causes of ARDS include all of the following EXCEPT

    A. multiple sclerosis
    B. multiple blood transfusions
    C. aspiration of gastric contents
    D. trauma and sepsis

11. It has been reported that inspiratory pressures greater than 70 cm H$_2$O are associated with a 43% risk of barotrauma.
    Risk factors for barotrauma include

    A. low residual volume
    B. large tidal volume
    C. low levels of PEEP
    D. low peak airway pressure

12. Barotrauma is the presence of air outside the alveolus and is manifested by
    I. pulmonary interstitial emphysema
    II. pneumomediastinum
    III. tension lung cysts
    The CORRECT answer is:

    A. I, II
    B. II only
    C. I, III
    D. I, II, III

13. The aim of therapy in a patient of ARDS is to support lung function until healing occurs and to prevent the development of complications related to medical therapy and the underlying disease process.
    Goals of therapeutic management include

    A. optimizing gas exchange
    B. maintaining adequate tissue perfusion
    C. controlling the underlying problem that precipitated ARDS
    D. all of the above

14. Nursing care for the patient with ARDS is planned to maintain respiratory and hemodynamic stability.
    Outcome criteria for the patient include all of the following EXCEPT

    A. PaO_2 below 60 mmHg on 40% FIO_2 with a shunt fraction of less than 20%
    B. peak airway pressure below 40-50 mmHg
    C. skin remains intact
    D. stable weight

15. Generally, mechanical ventilation of COPD patients is avoided if at all possible.
    Mechanical ventilation is NOT deemed necessary when

    A. conservative therapy has failed to improve hypoxemia/acidosis or has resulted in progressive somnolence
    B. the patient is exhausted
    C. the patient has severe hyperoxemia and alkalosis and is unable to cooperate because of altered mental status
    D. the patient is unable to expectorate secretions

16. The nursing care for COPD patients in acute respiratory failure is planned to achieve which of the following outcomes?

    A. Breathing pattern and arterial blood gas levels return to prefailure levels
    B. Lungs clear to auscultation
    C. Airway remains patent
    D. All of the above

17. Pneumonia is an inflammation of the lower respiratory tract that involves the lung parenchyma, including alveoli and supportive structures.
    The organism MOST commonly involved in the causation of community acquired pneumonia is

    A. klebsiella pneumonia
    B. staphylococcus aureus
    C. streptococcus pnemoniae
    D. pseudomonas aeruginosa

18. Hospital acquired, or nosocomial, pneumonias are LEAST commonly caused by   18.____

    A. pseudomonas aeruginosa   B. klebsiella pneumonia
    C. streptococcus pneumoniae   D. staphylococcus aureus

19. Which of the following persons are at INCREASED risk for aspiration pneumonia?   19.____
        I. Drug abusers
        II. Impaired gag or swallowing reflex
        III. Alcoholics
    The CORRECT answer is:

    A. I, II   B. I, II, III
    C. I, III   D. II only

20. Viral pneumonia in immunosuppressed patients is MOST commonly caused by   20.____

    A. cytomegalovirus
    B. influenza virus type A
    C. para influenza virus
    D. respiratory syncitial virus

21. Priorities for planning nursing care of patients with pneumonia include treatment of the   21.____
    infection, maintenance of adequate oxygenation, and maintenance of patent airways.
    While observing for evidence of complications, such as respiratory failure, appropriate
    outcome criteria include all of the following EXCEPT

    A. breath sounds clear with coughing
    B. PaO$_2$ less than 55 mmHg at rest and with activities
    C. sputum expectorated with minimal effort
    D. appetite returns to normal baseline

22. Tuberculosis can be highly contagious and is transmitted by airborne mechanisms from   22.____
    infected persons.
    The one of the following which is NOT a common cause of tuberculosis is

    A. mycobacterium tuberculosis
    B. M. bovis
    C. M. leprae
    D. M. africanum

23. Patients at INCREASED risk for drug-resistant tuberculosis include   23.____

    A. foreign-born persons from Asia, Africa, and Latin America
    B. persons with positive bacteriology after 3 months of therapy
    C. contacts of known or suspected drug-resistant cases
    D. all of the above

24. Lung cancer is a serious health problem in the United States.   24.____
    Risk factors for lung cancer include all of the following EXCEPT

    A. cigarette smoking
    B. amphetamine abuse
    C. asbestos exposure
    D. exposure to arsenic, radon, and chromium

25. Hematological manifestations associated with lung cancer include 25.____

   A. anemia
   B. disseminated intravascular coagulation
   C. thrombophlebitis
   D. all of the above

KEY (CORRECT ANSWERS)

1. C
2. B
3. D
4. A
5. C

6. B
7. C
8. A
9. C
10. A

11. B
12. D
13. D
14. A
15. C

16. D
17. C
18. C
19. B
20. A

21. B
22. C
23. D
24. B
25. D

EXAMINATION SECTION
TEST 1

DIRECTIONS: Each question or incomplete statement is followed by several suggested answers or completions. Select the one that BEST answers the question or completes the statement. *PRINT THE LETTER OF THE CORRECT ANSWER IN THE SPACE AT THE RIGHT.*

1. Radiation therapy is administered to selected patients with lung cancer. Toxic side effects of radiation therapy include

    A. esophagitis
    B. fibrosis
    C. pneumonitis
    D. all of the above

    1.____

2. The priority for nursing care of patients with lung cancer is maintenance of adequate gas exchange and airway clearance while trying to keep patients as comfortable as possible. For a patient in the acute phase, outcome criteria might include all of the following EXCEPT

    A. PaO_2 is less than 55 mmHg at rest and with activities
    B. sputum is expectorated with minimal effort
    C. patient maintains realistic level of activity
    D. patient sleeps comfortably at night and feels rested in the morning

    2.____

3. Nursing interventions for patients with dyspnea related to lung cancer should include

    A. relaxation techniques
    B. proper positioning and controlling the environment
    C. breathing techniques, such as pursed-lip breathing
    D. all of the above

    3.____

4. When a patient is admitted to the emergency room with chest trauma, the primary goal of nursing care is to maintain a patent airway, adequate ventilation, and adequate circulation while assessing the extent of injury. Outcome criteria for this patient include

    A. arterial PO_2 is maintained below 55 mmHg
    B. patient sleeps appropriate number of hours and reports feeling rested
    C. breath sounds are unclear with adventitious sounds
    D. patient reports maximal respiratory discomfort

    4.____

5. Atherosclerosis is the major pathologic process by which lipid deposits occur in the intimal and subintimal layers of the artery. *Controllable* risk factors for atherosclerosis include all of the following EXCEPT

    A. diabetes mellitus
    B. hyperlipidemia
    C. family history
    D. smoking

    5.____

6. Smoking is the most consistent risk factor in the literature on peripheral vascular occlusive disease.
Of the following, only _____ is NOT among the effects of smoking on the cardiovascular system.

    A. increased systolic blood pressure
    B. vasodilatation

    6.____

11

C. reduced exercise tolerance
D. increased heart rate

7. Effects of smoking on the blood include
   I. hemoconcentration
   II. decreased fibrinogen levels
   III. shorter platelet survival
   IV. decreased viscosity
   The CORRECT answer is:

   A. I, II
   B. I, III
   C. II, III, IV
   D. I, II, III, IV

8. The MOST common areas for developing atherosclerotic plaques include

   A. major arterial bifurcations
   B. aorta
   C. superficial femoral artery at Hunter's canal
   D. all of the above

9. Hyperlipidemia has been implicated in the development of arterial occlusive disease. Lipid effects as a result of smoking do NOT include increased

   A. total cholesterol
   B. HDL cholesterol
   C. permeability of vessels to lipids
   D. none of the above

10. Atherosclerosis is asymptomatic until a critical stenosis occurs in an artery. Effects of smoking on the blood vessels include all of the following EXCEPT

    A. decreased myointimal proliferation
    B. decreased oxygenation of vessel walls
    C. increased permeability of endothelium
    D. endothelial injury

11. Nursing management for the patient with atherosclerosis is planned so that the patient will

    A. adopt protective measures against injury of impaired tissue
    B. practice behavior to increase collateral circulation
    C. state the relationship between atherosclerosis and risk factors
    D. all of the above

12. Nursing interventions for patients with atherosclerosis are primarily for secondary and tertiary prevention.
    Patient education guidelines for antihyperlipidemic agents include all of the following EXCEPT

    A. mix medication with water or juice; do not take it dry
    B. take medication one hour before or 6 hours after other medications to avoid interference with absorption of other drugs
    C. do not take medications with meals
    D. report any gastrointestinal or other symptoms

13. An extranatomic bypass is a graft in the subcutaneous tissue instead of the abdominal cavity.
    High risk patients who may benefit from extranatomic bypass include all of the following EXCEPT those

    A. with intraabdominal infection or infected graft
    B. under 60 years of age
    C. with aortoenteric fistula present
    D. with morbid obesity

14. In the post-operative nursing care of a patient with a femoral-to-popliteal or femoral-to-distal tibial bypass graft, it is NOT necessary to

    A. assess the wound for bleeding or swelling from hematoma formation
    B. avoid flexing the groin or knees more than 45 degrees for extended periods
    C. allow the patient to put powder, lotion, or other materials in the groin to keep it wet
    D. avoid compression or circumferential dressings

15. The one of the following which is NOT among the goals of nursing management of a patient with chronic arterial occlusive disease of the extremities is that the patient

    A. manage activity within his own limits
    B. have minimum tissue perfusion
    C. have decreased pain
    D. practice self-care to avoid tissue damage

16. The operative mortality rate for elective aneurysm repair is approximately 5%, as opposed to 50-80% for the ruptured aneurysm.
    Post-operative nursing care of such a patient should include

    A. maintaining adequate fluid balance
    B. having adequate peripheral tissue perfusion
    C. having knowledge of discharge instructions
    D. all of the above

17. Raynaud's disease is the condition most often seen in patients with vasospastic disorders.
    Nursing care of a patient with Raynaud's disease aims to achieve

    A. demonstration of knowledge of measures to prevent recurrent episodes
    B. skin temperature, color, and pulse within patient's normal limits
    C. decreased number of episodes of arterial spasm
    D. all of the above

18. Patient education and emotional support are important aspects of nursing care.
    To avoid Raynaud's disease symptoms, patient education should include all of the following guidelines EXCEPT

    A. smoking cessation
    B. avoiding hot weather
    C. managing stress
    D. avoiding vibration

19. Thoracic outlet syndrome is a set of upper extremity symptoms resulting from neurovascular compression in the thoracic outlet area.
    These symptoms result from compression of the brachial nerve plexus and the subclavian artery and vein by all of the following structures EXCEPT the

    A. scalenus posterior muscles
    B. clavicle
    C. scalenus anterior muscles
    D. first rib

20. A nurse is teaching a patient about thoracic outlet syndromes.
    It is TRUE concerning the nursing care of this patient that the

    A. overweight patient won't benefit from a weight reduction plan
    B. nurse can reinforce the exercise program and refer the patient to physical therapy
    C. nurse may also provide emotional and financial support to the patient
    D. all of the above

21. In the past, medications have been the major mode of therapy for patients with hypertension. Greater emphasis is now being placed on nonpharmacologic approaches by the National Committee on Hypertension.
    These nonpharmacological approaches do NOT include

    A. sodium restriction   B. restricted water intake
    C. weight control   D. alcohol restriction

22. Vasodilators used in the treatment of hypertension act by decreasing peripheral vascular resistance. Their side effects include all of the following EXCEPT

    A. headaches   B. orthostatic hypotension
    C. bronchospasm   D. fluid retention

23. Six criteria have been established by the Joint National Committee on Detection, Evaluation, and Treatment of Hypertension to ensure accurate blood pressure measurement.
    Of the following, the INCORRECT statement is:

    A. Patient should be in a lying down position with arm positioned above heart level
    B. Measurement should begin after 5 minutes of quiet rest
    C. Appropriate cuff size must be used to ensure accurate measurement
    D. Both the systolic and diastolic blood pressures should be recorded

24. The decision to begin anti-hypertensive therapy is usually a lifetime commitment for a patient. It is imperative that the nurse, as the patient's advocate and educator, answer the patient's questions thoroughly before the patient engages in therapy.
    Subjects for the nurse to evaluate include

    A. age: young people have higher renin levels than older ones
    B. weight: excessive weight tends to occur with increasing age
    C. level of blood pressure: mild hypertension may be treated nonpharmacologically
    D. all of the above

25. Cardiopulmonary arrest in the hospital setting commonly results in a *Code* situation. 25.____
In a code situation, someone from the team is usually REQUIRED to
   I. manage the airway and IV access
   II. perform chest compressions
   III. document all activities
The CORRECT answer is:

A. I, II
B. II, III
C. I, II, III
D. III *only*

KEY (CORRECT ANSWERS)

1. D
2. A
3. D
4. B
5. C

6. B
7. B
8. D
9. B
10. A

11. D
12. C
13. B
14. C
15. B

16. D
17. D
18. B
19. A
20. B

21. B
22. C
23. A
24. D
25. C

TEST 2

DIRECTIONS: Each question or incomplete statement is followed by several suggested answers or completions. Select the one that BEST answers the question or completes the statement. *PRINT THE LETTER OF THE CORRECT ANSWER IN THE SPACE AT THE RIGHT.*

1. Approximately 50,000 to 60,000 people in the United States die each year from pulmonary emboli that originate from deep vein thrombosis (DVT).
   Disease processes that predispose the patient to DVT include all of the following EXCEPT

   A. congenital heart failure
   B. tuberculosis
   C. sepsis
   D. myocardial infarction

   1.____

2. A nurse taking care of a patient with deep vein thrombosis should instruct the patient to

   A. take anticoagulant at a different time each day
   B. take aspirin or ibuprofen
   C. use soft brush and electric razor
   D. all of the above

   2.____

3. A nurse is assessing a patient for risk factors for deep vein thrombosis and pulmonary embolism.
   Patient instruction should include all of the following advice EXCEPT:

   A. Do not sit or cross legs for prolonged periods
   B. If traveling, exercise at least every 12 hours
   C. Do not wear constrictive clothing
   D. Know the classic signs of pulmonary embolism

   3.____

4. Atrial tachycardia describes an ectopic supraventricular rhythm with a ventricular rate ranging from 140 to 250 beats per minute.
   ECG criteria for diagnosis do NOT include

   A. P'-P' interval may be slightly irregular
   B. ectopic P waves look alike and closely resemble sinus P waves
   C. QRS is wide unless intraventricular conduction is disturbed
   D. P'R interval is short

   4.____

5. Atrioventricular blocks (AVBs) represent disturbed conduction of the electrical impulse between the atria and ventricles.
   AVBs may be produced in association with all of the following EXCEPT

   A. reduced vagal tone
   B. myocardial ischemia
   C. electrolyte imbalances
   D. compression of conduction tissue

   5.____

6. A pacemaker is an electronic device that delivers a controlled electrical stimulus to the heart through electrodes that are placed in contact with heart muscles. Permanent pacing is indicated in cases of
   I. mild palpitations
   II. sick sinus syndrome
   III. myocardial necrosis
   The CORRECT answer is:

   A. I, II
   B. I *only*
   C. I, II, III
   D. II, III

   6.____

7. Congestive heart failure represents the inability of the heart to pump enough blood to meet tissue requirements for oxygen.
   Primary pathologic conditions associated with acute and chronic forms of heart failure include

   A. hypertension
   B. valvular heart diseases
   C. cardiomyopathies
   D. all of the above

   7.____

8. The signs and symptoms of heart failure reflect the status of intrinsic compensatory mechanisms and vary according to the degree of failure.
   Physiologic, endocrine, and renal responses to heart failure include

   A. decreased antidiuretic hormone
   B. decreased glomerular filtration rate
   C. decreased aldosterone
   D. increased urinary output

   8.____

9. Nursing advice for patients of coronary artery disease concerning the avoidance of activities that may increase myocardial oxygen demand include all of the following EXCEPT

   A. avoid excessive caffeine intake
   B. be sure to get enough physical activity after meals
   C. avoid activities known to cause anginal pain, e.g., extremes of temperature, exertion, and attitudes
   D. avoid alcohol

   9.____

10. Myocardial infarction (MI) is an acute process in which myocardial tissues experience a severe and prolonged decrease in oxygen supply because of a disruption or deficiency in coronary blood flow, causing necrosis or *death* of the tissue.
    Of the following, only _____ is NOT among the causes of MI.

    A. acute coronary thrombosis
    B. amphetamine abuse
    C. coronary artery spasm
    D. cocaine abuse

    10.____

11. A patient of MI is discharged from the hospital.
    Nursing advice for the progression of activities for this patient should include all of the following EXCEPT

    A. increase activity level gradually
    B. avoid lifting heavy objects, isometric activities, straining, or pushing

    11.____

C. eat two or three large meals rather than several small meals per day
D. ensure adequate sleep with daily rest periods

12. In a case of myocardial infarction, activity progression is based on the patient's physiologic response.
Activity tolerance is determined using which of the following criteria?

    A. Heart rate increase less than 20 beats/minute
    B. No decrease in systolic blood pressure
    C. No chest pain, dyspnea, extreme fatigue, or dysrhythmias
    D. All of the above

13. When instructing a discharging patient of MI, the nurse should tell him to report IMMEDIATELY if he experiences

    A. increased shortness of breath
    B. rapid weight gain
    C. dizziness or fainting
    D. all of the above

14. Pericarditis refers to an inflammation of the pericardium, the membrane surrounding the heart. Autoimmune causes of pericarditis include all of the following EXCEPT

    A. tuberculosis
    B. Dressier's syndrome
    C. rheumatic disease
    D. systemic lupus erythematosus

15. Dilated cardiomyopathy is a disorder of the myocardium characterized by impaired contractility and pumping ability.
Its precipitating factors do NOT include

    A. immunologic disorders
    B. pregnancy
    C. uncontrolled hypotension
    D. chronic alcohol ingestion

16. Nursing goals for patients must be tailored to meet the needs of each individual, considering the type of cardiomyopathy and the age, social setting, and severity of illness of the patient. Goals for the patient aim to ensure that

    A. patient can tolerate mild activity and build activity into each day
    B. respirations are comfortable and breath sounds are clear
    C. anxiety is channeled constructively, with reduction in stress
    D. all of the above

17. When cardiac surgery is performed for coronary artery obstruction, a coronary artery bypass graft (CABG) is used.
All of the following complications may occur as a result of cardiac surgery or the use of a cardiopulmonary bypass machine EXCEPT

    A. hyperthermia   B. coagulation defects
    C. hemodilution   D. reduced lung compliance

18. Infective endocarditis is an infection of the endocardial layer of the heart. Infecting bacterial causes include

    A. staphylococcus aureus
    B. pseudomonas
    C. enterococcus
    D. all of the above

18.____

19. Sickle cell anemia is a disorder of abnormal hemoglobin, also termed hemoglobinopathy, in which one or both of the polypeptide chains are abnormal.
    Management of pain episodes associated with sickle cell anemia include all of the following EXCEPT

    A. cold application to joints
    B. analgesics
    C. rest
    D. hydration

19.____

20. Chronic mitral regurgitation, also known as mitral insufficiency, is often seen with mitral stenosis. Rheumatic heart disease is the predominant cause.
    Other causes of mitral regurgitation include

        I. infective endocarditis
        II. mitral valve prolapse
        III. leakage through a prosthetic valve

    The CORRECT answer is:

    A. I, II
    B. II *only*
    C. I, II, III
    D. II, III

20.____

21. Because such a large number of elderly people are affected by a vitamin B_{12} deficiency, causing megaloblastic anemia, it is important to assess the elderly in this area. This is particularly important since this deficiency may not be diagnosed because older adults frequently attribute signs of deficiency to age and do not seek medical assistance. Signs and symptoms of vitamin B_{12} deficiency include all of the following EXCEPT

    A. sore and beefy tongue
    B. osteoarthritis
    C. paranoia
    D. numbness and tingling peripherally

21.____

22. Leukemia is a group of malignant diseases of the bone marrow and is characterized by an unregulated proliferation of cells of hematopoietic origin.
    Predisposing genetic abnormalities for leukemia include all of the following EXCEPT

    A. Down's syndrome
    B. fragile *X* syndrome
    C. Fanconi's anemia
    D. Wiskott-Aldrich's syndrome

22.____

23. Tumor lysis syndrome is a major complication of chemotherapy in acute lymphocytic leukemia.
    The one of the following which is NOT a complication of tumor lysis syndrome is

    A. hypokalemia
    B. hyperphosphatemia
    C. hypocalcemia
    D. hyperuricemia

23.____

24. Multiple myeloma is a neoplastic proliferation of plasma cells, characterized by lytic bone lesions, anemia, and homogeneous serum or urinary globulin elevation. Nursing interventions in this case aims to do all of the following EXCEPT

    A. prevent infection
    B. keep patient immobile
    C. provide pain relief
    D. provide adequate hydration

25. Disseminated intravascular coagulation (DIC) is an acquired syndrome of clotting cascade overstimulation. Predisposing hematological causes of DIC do NOT include

    A. blood transfusion reaction
    B. sickle cell crisis
    C. iron deficiency anemia
    D. thalassemia major

KEY (CORRECT ANSWERS)

1.	B	11.	C
2.	C	12.	D
3.	B	13.	D
4.	C	14.	A
5.	A	15.	C
6.	D	16.	D
7.	D	17.	A
8.	B	18.	D
9.	B	19.	A
10.	B	20.	C

21.	B
22.	B
23.	A
24.	B
25.	C

EXAMINATION SECTION
TEST 1

DIRECTIONS: Each question or incomplete statement is followed by several suggested answers or completions. Select the one that BEST answers the question or completes the statement. *PRINT THE LETTER OF THE CORRECT ANSWER IN THE SPACE AT THE RIGHT.*

Questions 1-2.

DIRECTIONS: Questions 1 and 2 are to be answered on the basis of the following information.

Mrs. Smith, 34 years old, is admitted to the hospital after an automobile accident. She has a fractured hip and is taken to surgery for repair. On return from surgery, Mrs. Smith is very much concerned about her obesity.

1. Mrs. Smith asks the nurse how she should lose weight. The nurse's BEST reply would be to tell her that 1.____

    A. fats should be limited in her diet
    B. she needs to exercise vigorously no matter what she eats
    C. her eating pattern should be altered with all 4 basic groups and include light exercise
    D. only carbohydrates have to be completely stopped

2. The physician ordered non-weight bearing with crutches for Mrs. Smith. 2.____
What should the nurse advise her regarding walking with crutches?

    A. To strengthen the muscles, exercise them, using triceps, finger flexors, and elbow extensors
    B. Sitting up in a chair strengthens back muscles
    C. The head and neck muscles should be exercised
    D. None of the above

Questions 3-7.

DIRECTIONS: Questions 3 through 7 are to be answered on the basis of the following information.

John, a factory worker, is admitted to the hospital for mild chest pain. A myocardial infarct is diagnosed. The physician orders morphine sulphate, diazepam, and lidocaine.

3. John asks the nurse why he is being given morphine sulphate. 3.____
The nurse should tell him that morphine sulphate

    A. relieves pain associated with myocardial infarction
    B. decreases apprehension
    C. prevents cardiogenic shock
    D. all of the above

4. The patient is also prescribed oxygen by nasal cannula. The nurse takes safety precautions in the room because oxygen

   A. converts to an alternate form of matter
   B. supports combustion
   C. has unstable properties
   D. is flammable

5. In a case of myocardial infarction, the finding on the electrocardiogram should be

   A. disappearance of Q waves
   B. absent P wave
   C. elevated ST segments
   D. flattened T waves

6. Several days after admission, John develops pyrexia.
   The nurse should monitor him for

   A. dyspnea
   B. increased pulse rate
   C. chest pain
   D. elevated blood pressure

7. John asks the nurse about the chances of his having another heart attack if he watches his diet and stress level.
   The nurse should

   A. tell him he is at no risk
   B. suggest that he talk to a psychiatric nurse for his fear about this
   C. avoid giving him direct information
   D. none of the above

Questions 8-10.

DIRECTIONS: Questions 8 through 10 are to be answered on the basis of the following information.

Mrs. Allbright is 65 years old and is suspected to have pernicious anemia.

8. The first test ordered is a Schillings test.
   The nurse should know that the purpose of this test is to check the person's ability to _____ vitamin B _____.

   A. absorb; 12
   B. digest; 12
   C. absorb; 6
   D. store; 1

9. The nurse should explain the therapeutic regimen for pernicious anemia to Mrs. Allbright as consisting of

   A. oral tablets of B_{12} daily
   B. IM injections daily
   C. IM injections once a month
   D. oral tablets every week

10. Mrs. Allbright wants to know how long she will need therapy. 10.____
    The nurse should reply that she will need therapy

    A. when she feels fatigued
    B. for the rest of her life
    C. until her symptoms subside
    D. during exacerbations of anemia

Questions 11-16.

DIRECTIONS: Questions 11 through 16 are to be answered on the basis of the following information.

Mr. Roberts is 45 years old. He is brought to the emergency room after a terrible motor vehicle accident in which he received multiple crushing wounds of the chest, abdomen, and legs. His right leg might have to be amputated.

11. Upon arrival, the nursing staff's FIRST priority should be to assess 11.____

    A. blood pressure
    B. pain
    C. quality of respiration and presence of pulse
    D. level of consciousness

12. Mr. Roberts' condition requires endotracheal intubation and positive pressure ventilation. 12.____
    The IMMEDIATE nursing intervention should be to

    A. facilitate verbal communication
    B. assess his response to the equipment
    C. maintain sterility of ventilation system
    D. prepare for emergency surgery

13. A chest tube with water seal drainage is inserted. The chest tube seems obstructed. 13.____
    The MOST appropriate nursing action at this time would be to

    A. clamp tube immediately
    B. remove chest tube
    C. milk the tube toward collection container
    D. take a chest x-ray

14. What is the function of the chest tube placed in Mr. Roberts? 14.____
    To

    A. normalize intrathoracic pressure
    B. drain fluid from pleural space
    C. drain air from pleural space
    D. all of the above

15. A response that would indicate that Mr. Roberts' condition was improving is 15.____

    A. increased breath sounds
    B. constant bubbling in drainage chamber
    C. increased respiratory rate
    D. crepitus on palpation of chest

16. In Mr. Roberts' case, adequate tissue perfusion to vital organs would be indicated by   16.____

    A. central venous pressure of 2 cm H$_2$O
    B. urinary output of 30 ml in an hour
    C. pulse rate of 120-110 in 15 minutes
    D. blood pressure of 50/30 and 70/40 in 30 minutes

17. A 47-year-old man is brought into the emergency room following an accident. He has   17.____
    severe abdominal pain in the left upper quadrant. Splenic rupture is diagnosed, and an
    emergency splenectomy is to be performed.
    The nurse should tell the patient

    A. about the presence of abdominal drains several days after surgery
    B. that splenectomy has a low mortality rate (5%), except with multiple injuries
    C. not to worry about bleeding as it occurs more frequently with repairs than removal
    D. all of the above

Questions 18-19.

DIRECTIONS: Questions 18 and 19 are to be answered on the basis of the following information.

A 34-year-old woman was involved in an accident as a result of which her left leg had to be amputated below the knee. After the operation, the patient refused to talk, eat, or perform any activities.

18. The BEST nursing approach in this case would be to   18.____

    A. appear cheerful, regardless of the patient's condition
    B. force her to do exercises
    C. accept and acknowledge that withdrawal is an initially normal and necessary part of grieving
    D. emphasize that nothing has changed in her life and she can and should resume normal life

19. The factors responsible for this change in this patient include the _____ of the change.   19.____

    A. client's perception   B. suddenness
    C. extent   D. all of the above

20. In dealing with a terminally ill patient who is in the denial stage of grief, the BEST nursing   20.____
    approach is to

    A. encourage the patient's denial
    B. reassure the patient that everything will be okay
    C. allow denial but be available to discuss death
    D. leave the patient alone

Questions 21-25.

DIRECTIONS: Questions 21 through 25 are to be answered on the basis of the following information

A 62-year-old patient is admitted to the coronary care unit with a diagnosis of left-sided congestive heart failure.

21. The findings in this case would MOST likely include

    A. dyspnea on exertion
    B. chest pain of the crushing type
    C. peripheral edema
    D. jugular vein distention

22. This patient was ordered a cardiac glycoside, a vasodilator, and furosemide (lasix). The site of effect of furosemide is the

    A. collecting tube
    B. ascending loop of Henle
    C. distil tube
    D. glomerulus

23. The distil tube is the site of action of

    A. thiazides
    B. triamtere
    C. xanthines
    D. spironolactone

24. Cardiac glycosides, such as digitalis, _____ the conduction speed in the myocardium and _____ the heart rate.

    A. increase; slow down
    B. increase; speed up
    C. decrease; slow down
    D. decrease; speed up

25. In cases of congestive heart failure, the nurse should suggest a dietary restriction of

    A. potassium   B. sodium   C. magnesium   D. iron

KEY (CORRECT ANSWERS)

1. C	11. C
2. A	12. B
3. D	13. C
4. B	14. D
5. C	15. A
6. B	16. B
7. C	17. D
8. A	18. C
9. C	19. D
10. B	20. C

21. A
22. B
23. A
24. C
25. B

TEST 2

DIRECTIONS: Each question or incomplete statement is followed by several suggested answers or completions. Select the one that BEST answers the question or completes the statement. *PRINT THE LETTER OF THE CORRECT ANSWER IN THE SPACE AT THE RIGHT.*

1. While taking a history of a patient with G.I. bleeding, the nurse should put the MOST emphasis on

    A. family history
    B. socioeconomic history
    C. history of any recent medications such as aspirin or prednisone
    D. travel of an endemic area

    1.____

2. What kind of dietary management is APPROPRIATE for a patient with gastric ulceration to prevent the mucosal lining from the adverse effects of acids?

    A. Three meals a day
    B. Regular meals and snacks to relieve gastric discomfort
    C. One meal a day
    D. Eat whenever hungry

    2.____

3. Precautions that should be taken by a nurse in order to prevent infections from an indwelling catheter include

    A. changing the bag periodically and not emptying it
    B. maintaining the ordered hydration which flushes the bladder and prevents infection
    C. collecting specimens in order to check for infection
    D. all of the above

    3.____

Questions 4-7.

DIRECTIONS: Questions 4 through 7 are to be answered on the basis of the following information.

Mr. Connery, a 65-year-old patient, is scheduled for surgery of transurethral resection of the prostate.

4. The nurse should let Mr. Connery know that after surgery

    A. his urinary control may be completely lost
    B. urinary drainage will be by a catheter for 24-48 hours
    C. everything will be completely normal
    D. his ability to perform sexually will be completely impaired

    4.____

5. In Mr. Connery's case, the MOST common complication following surgery is

    A. hemorrhage
    B. sepsis
    C. urinary retention with overflow
    D. none of the above

    5.____

2 (#2)

6. 24 hours after surgery, Mr. Connery, who is still on a catheter, complains of lower abdominal discomfort. The nurse notices that catheter drainage has stopped.
   The nurse's NEXT step should be to

   A. remove the catheter
   B. notify the physician
   C. irrigate with saline
   D. milk the catheter tubing

6._____

7. Which of the following discharge instructions given by the nurse is MOST important for Mr. Connery?

   A. Void at least every 3 hours
   B. Avoid exercise for 6 months after surgery
   C. Call the physician if urinary stream decreases
   D. Get 18 hours of sleep every 24 hours

7._____

Questions 8-10.

DIRECTIONS: Questions 8 through 10 are to be answered on the basis of the following information.

Mrs. Ford is admitted to the hospital for a subtotal thyroidectomy. She has a history of Grave's disease.

8. It is important that the nurse know that in a subtotal thyroidectomy

   A. the entire thyroid gland is removed
   B. a small part is left intact
   C. part of the parathyroid is also removed
   D. only parathyroids are removed

8._____

9. Classical signs of hyperthyroidism include

   A. weight loss
   C. restlessness
   B. exopthalmos
   D. all of the above

9._____

10. Signs of postsurgical hypothyroidism of which Mrs. Ford should be aware include

    A. intolerance to heat
    C. dry skin and fatigue
    B. weight loss
    D. insomnia

10._____

Questions 11-13.

DIRECTIONS: Questions 11 through 13 are to be answered on the basis of the following information.

Lisa, a 32-year-old woman, is admitted for treatment of partial and full thickness burns on the lower half of her body. She is in pain.

11. The nurse applies sulphamylon cream to Lisa's burns. This will

    A. relieve the pain
    B. inhibit bacterial growth

11._____

C. provide debridement
D. prevent scar tissue formation

12. Pig skin temporary grafts are used for Lisa's burns. The grafts will

    A. relieve the pain
    B. promote rapid epethelialization
    C. provide a framework for granulation
    D. all of the above

13. Lisa suffers from periodic episodes of dyspnea.
    The BEST position for her is the _____ position.

    A. orthopheic   B. sims
    C. semi-fowler's   D. supine

Questions 14-17.

DIRECTIONS: Questions 14 through 17 are to be answered on the basis of the following information.

Mrs. Hunt is 61 years old. She has a history of hypertension over the past 15 years. She complains of dyspnea and pedal edema.

14. The dyspnea is PROBABLY due to

    A. asthma
    B. left ventricular failure
    C. wheezing and coughing
    D. none of the above

15. Mrs. Hunt has been prescribed hydrochlorothiazide.
    A COMMON side effect of this drug is

    A. insomnia
    B. increased thirst
    C. generalized weakness due to hypokalemia
    D. increased muscle strength as a result of hypercalcemia

16. Mrs. Hunt has also been prescribed a potassium supplement because of the diuretic she is taking.
    Potassium supplements

    A. are completely harmless
    B. should not be taken on an empty stomach as they cause GI ulceration and bleeding
    C. possess no side effects at all
    D. all of the above

17. The nurse should tell Mrs. Hunt to

    A. rest during the day to decrease the demand on her heart
    B. sleep with her head slightly elevated to facilitate respiration

C. take her pulse just once daily
D. all of the above

Questions 18-20.

DIRECTIONS: Questions 18 through 20 are to be answered on the basis of the following information.

Mr. Edwards had a partial nephrectomy done and is admitted with a nephrostomy tube in place.

18. The MOST common life-threatening complication in the early post-operative period is   18.____

    A. sepsis   B. hemorrhage
    C. renal failure   D. none of the above

19. The nurse's post-operative plan for Mr. Edwards should include   19.____

    A. turning him from back to operated site to facilitate drainage
    B. keeping him on clear fluid for 24-48 hours
    C. draining dressing frequently
    D. all of the above

20. Upon discharge, Mr. Edwards, who is being discharged with nephrostomy tube in place, should be instructed to   20.____

    A. change dressings frequently
    B. limit fluid intake
    C. maintain bedrest at home
    D. all of the above

21. Mrs. Beatty comes to the clinic with complaints of increased appetite, thirst, and weight loss despite more eating. She is diagnosed with diabetes mellitus, and the doctor prescribed her an oral hypoglycemic.
    The MOST common side effect of oral hypoglycemic agents is   21.____

    A. diabetic coma   B. weight loss
    C. hypoglycemia   D. all of the above

Questions 22-25.

DIRECTIONS: Questions 22 through 25 are to be answered on the basis of the following information.

Mr. Mailer, a 34-year-old executive, is diagnosed with a peptic ulcer.

22. The pain of a peptic ulcer is COMMONLY described as   22.____

    A. dull pain in the shoulder
    B. gnawing and boring in the epigastrium and back
    C. sharp pain in the abdomen
    D. heartburn upon lying down

23. The physician prescribes ranitidine for Mr. Mailer. Ranitidine   23._____

    A. can be given PO, IV, or IM
    B. is usually given with meals
    C. reduces gastric acid in the stomach
    D. all of the above

24. Mr. Mailer's condition worsens while in the hospital. He vomited and complained of   24._____
    severe epigastric pain. His pulse is 134, respiration is 32/minute, and there is an
    absence of bowel sounds. The nurse calls for the physician.
    The NEXT step should be to

    A. keep the client NPO in preparation for possible surgery
    B. start oxygen
    C. place the client in the Trendelenberg position
    D. all of the above

25. A subtotal gastrectomy (Billroth 1) is performed on Mr. Mailer. He starts eating more   25._____
    food, but he experiences cramping discomfort and rapid pulse with waves of weakness
    followed by nausea and vomiting.
    The nurse recognizes that Mr. Mailer is going through a *dumping syndrome* caused by
    the _____ into the small intestine.

    A. slow passage of food dumping
    B. rapid passage of food (hyperosmolar)
    C. rapid passage of dilute food
    D. none of the above

KEY (CORRECT ANSWERS)

1.	C		11.	B
2.	B		12.	D
3.	D		13.	A
4.	B		14.	B
5.	A		15.	C
6.	D		16.	B
7.	C		17.	D
8.	B		18.	B
9.	D		19.	D
10.	C		20.	A

21. C
22. B
23. D
24. A
25. B

EXAMINATION SECTION
TEST 1

DIRECTIONS: Each question or incomplete statement is followed by several suggested answers or completions. Select the one that BEST answers the question or completes the statement. *PRINT THE LETTER OF THE CORRECT ANSWER IN THE SPACE AT THE RIGHT.*

Questions 1-3.

DIRECTIONS: Questions 1 through 3 are to be answered on the basis of the following information.

Anna comes in with a variety of vague complaints over the past 8 months. The physician suspects multiple sclerosis.

1. The MOST common initial symptom associated with multiple sclerosis is

   A. diplopia; blurred vision
   B. diarrhea
   C. dementia
   D. dermatitis

2. Anna, when the diagnosis of MS is confirmed, feels very upset and asks if she is going to die.
   The nurse should reply:

   A. Most individuals live a normal life span
   B. Ask the doctor
   C. Everyone has to die one day
   D. Prognosis is variable with remissions and exacerbations

3. Anna complains of urinary urgency and frequency.
   What should be the INITIAL nursing measure?

   A. Palpatate the supra pubic area to assess if the symptoms are caused by a full bladder
   B. Monitor urinary output
   C. Limit fluids
   D. All of the above

Questions 4-5.

DIRECTIONS: Questions 4 and 5 are to be answered on the basis of the following information.
Mary fractured her left hip as a result of falling on the doorstep. A fractured hip and osteoporosis are confirmed by x-ray.

4. The change in the x-ray due to osteoporosis which is MOST easily observable is

   A. compression fractures of vertebrae   B. long bones
   C. facial bones   D. joints of hands and feet

5. In order to limit the further progression of osteoporosis, the nurse should advise Mary to

   A. increase consumption of milk
   B. take supplemental calcium and vitamin D
   C. increase consumption of eggs
   D. take supplemental vitamin E

Questions 6-11.

DIRECTIONS: Questions 6 through 11 are to be answered on the basis of the following information.

Mr. Thompson is admitted for diagnosis and treatment of a lesion in the right lung. A bronchoscopy is performed.

6. The nurse should withhold food and fluids for several hours to prevent

   A. abdominal pain
   B. dyspepsia
   C. dysphagia
   D. aspiration of food

7. Mr. Thompson is diagnosed with lung cancer, and pneumonec-tomy is performed. The physician orders IV fluids at 80 ml/hour.
   To adjust the drip rate, the nurse must know the

   A. drops per milliliter delivered by the infusion set-up
   B. total volume in the IV bag
   C. diameter of tubing used
   D. size of needle or catheter in vein

8. On the first post-operative day, Mr. Thompson suddenly sits up in bed. His respiration is labored, and he is making a crowing sound. He seems very pale.
   The nurse should

   A. notify the physician
   B. auscultate the left lung
   C. check the tube for patency
   D. provide warm blankets

9. The BEST position that Mr. Thompson can use for lying which would permit good ventilation is the _____ position.

   A. supine or right lying
   B. supine or left lying
   C. Fowler's
   D. all of the above

10. Irradiation is prescribed for Mr. Thompson on an outpatient basis.
    The nurse should tell Mr. Thompson how to take care of his skin and should EMPHASIZE

    A. frequent washings
    B. massaging 4-7 times to increase circulation
    C. keeping skin dry and protecting from abrasions
    D. all of the above

11. In order to prevent vitamin D toxicity, Mr. Thompson should AVOID eating 11.____

    A. fruit and eggnog
    B. cottage cheese
    C. milk products and whole milk
    D. all of the above

12. _____ are at INCREASED risk for developing gall bladder disease. 12.____

    A. Females under age 40 with a family history of gallstones
    B. Males under age 40 with a past history of hepatitis
    C. Females over age 40 who are obese
    D. Males over age 40 who have low serum cholesterol

13. Which of the following is TRUE regarding an oral chole-cystogram done for a diagnosis 13.____
    of gallstones?

    A. The test is given on 1 day and it must be repeated if the results are inconclusive.
    B. A low fat dinner is given so that large amounts of bile will be stored in the gallbladder on the day of the test.
    C. The contrast medium in the pills often causes diarrhea.
    D. All of the above

14. The MOST important dietary modification in a patient before cholecystectomy is to be 14.____
    performed is

    A. eating low cholesterol foods to avoid formation of gallstones
    B. eating soft-textured foods to aid digestion
    C. reducing fats to avoid stimulation of the cholecysto-kinin mechanism for bile release
    D. increasing proteins to promote tissue healing

Questions 15-19.

DIRECTIONS: Questions 15 through 19 are to be answered on the basis of the following information.

   Mr. Dillon is admitted to the hospital for a fever of unknown origin. He recently experienced an unexplained weight loss and a series of respiratory infections. Mr. Dillon is accompanied by Mr. Jordan, who is his life partner. AIDS-related complex is suspected.

15. An AIDS diagnosis is based on a positive HIV antibody test and 15.____

    A. a history of weight loss
    B. a history of very high fevers
    C. the presence of an associated opportunistic infection
    D. a positive ELISA test

16. When taking Mr. Dillon's blood pressure, the nurse MUST

    A. wear gloves
    B. wear mask and gown
    C. wash hands thoroughly
    D. none of the above

17. Mr. Dillon is receiving AZT.
    The MOST important thing for the nurse to monitor is

    A. complete blood cell count
    B. serum electrolytes
    C. cardiac enzymes
    D. liver enzymes

18. It is important for the nurse to monitor complete blood count for Mr. Dillon because AZT causes

    A. anemia
    B. leukopenia
    C. granulocytopenia
    D. all of the above

19. The difference between AIDS and AIDS-related complex (ARC) is that ARC is

    A. more physiologically debilitating
    B. not transmitted by blood contact
    C. not associated with opportunistic infection
    D. not infective to other persons

Questions 20-25.

DIRECTIONS: Questions 20 through 25 are to be answered on the basis of the following information.

Mr. Burton is admitted to the hospital with severe left flank pain, nausea, and hematuria. Ureteral calculus is suspected.

20. What should be the FIRST nursing action after admission?

    A. Increase fluid intake
    B. Administer prescribed analgesics
    C. Obtain urine for urinalysis
    D. Obtain urine for culture and sensitivity

21. The type of pain MOST likely described by Mr. Burton to lead to a diagnosis of ureteral calculus is

    A. boring pain in the flank
    B. pain intensified on micturation
    C. spasmodic pain on the left side radiating to the suprapubis
    D. constant pain in the costovertebral angle

22. To prepare for an intravenous pyelogram to be done the next morning, the nurse should advise Mr. Burton to

    A. omit dinner the night before
    B. take a laxative before going to bed
    C. take a fat-free dinner
    D. stop all liquids

23. The intravenous pyelogram confirmed the presence of a stone. 23._____
 If Mr. Burton's blood test indicated elevated purine instead of calcium, then the stone would PROBABLY be composed of

    A. struvite
    B. oxalate
    C. cystine
    D. uric acid

24. By the next day, Mr. Burton's urinary output is much less than his intake. 24._____
 If his bladder is NOT distended, then the nurse should suspect

    A. oliguria
    B. renal failure
    C. hydroureter
    D. all of the above

25. A ureterolithotomy was performed on Mr. Burton. 25._____
 Signs and symptoms of urinary tract infections of which Mr. Burton should be made aware before being discharged include

    A. urgency and frequency of urination
    B. burning on urination
    C. fever
    D. all of the above

KEY (CORRECT ANSWERS)

1.	A	11.	D
2.	D	12.	C
3.	A	13.	D
4.	A	14.	C
5.	B	15.	C
6.	D	16.	C
7.	A	17.	A
8.	B	18.	D
9.	A	19.	C
10.	C	20.	B

21. C
22. B
23. D
24. C
25. D

TEST 2

DIRECTIONS: Each question or incomplete statement is followed by several suggested answers or completions. Select the one that BEST answers the question or completes the statement. *PRINT THE LETTER OF THE CORRECT ANSWER IN THE SPACE AT THE RIGHT.*

Questions 1-2.

DIRECTIONS: Questions 1 and 2 are to be answered on the basis of the following information.

Mr. Wilson, who has a 25-year history of excessive alcohol consumption, is admitted to the hospital with jaundice and acites.

1. What nursing action is MOST important in the first 48 hours after admission?

    A. Increase fluid intake
    B. Improve nutritional status
    C. Monitor vital signs
    D. Prepare for rehabilitative therapy

2. Mr. Wilson complains of severe pruritis.
   In order to relieve this, the physician would PROBABLY suggest

    A. sponge baths with alcohol
    B. application of baby oil
    C. application of cold cream
    D. baths with sodium bicarbonate solution

3. The typical gait associated with Parkinson's disease is referred to as

    A. ataxic   B. spastic
    C. scissoring   D. shuffling

4. While performing a physical examination and taking the history of a patient of Parkinson's disease, the nurse should assess the patient for

    A. hyperextension of the neck
    B. low-pitched, monotonous voice
    C. frequent bouts of diarrhea
    D. recent increase in appetite

5. Common signs and symptoms of Parkinson's disease include

    A. characteristic masked facies
    B. non-intention tremor
    C. constipation
    D. all of the above

6. Side effects related to levodopa include

    A. anorexia   B. tachycardia
    C. nausea   D. all of the above

7. In patients receiving heparin therapy, there is always potential for hemorrhage. The nurse in such a case should be ready to administer

   A. vitamin K
   B. warfarin
   C. protamine sulphate
   D. panheparin

Questions 8-11.

DIRECTIONS: Questions 8 through 11 are to be answered on the basis of the following information.

Mr. Foster is admitted to the hospital for repair of bilateral inguinal hernias under general anesthesia.

8. Before surgery, the nurse should look for signs of strangulation of hernias. An EARLY sign of strangulation would be

   A. projectile vomiting
   B. sharp abdominal pain
   C. increased flatus
   D. decreased bowel sounds

9. Pre-operatively, the nurse should teach Mr. Foster how to _____, as he will have to do it post-operatively.

   A. perform coughing and deep breathing exercises
   B. turn and change his position every 2 hours
   C. have a nasogastric tube in his nose
   D. all of the above

10. After the bilateral herniorrhaphy, Mr. Foster should be observed for the development of

    A. a hydrocele
    B. urinary retention
    C. paralytic ileus
    D. thrombophlebitis

11. If Mr. Foster's scrotum becomes swollen, the nurse should

    A. assist him with a sitz bath
    B. apply warm soaks to the scrotum
    C. prepare for incision and drainage
    D. elevate the scrotum using soft support

12. Mrs. McDonald, a 62-year-old obese woman, comes in complaining of being tired all the time. Her tests reveal hyperglycemia. She is diagnosed with type II diabetes. The nurse should expect Mrs. McDonald's lab values to reveal

    A. ketones in blood but not in urine
    B. urine negative for ketones but 4+ glucose
    C. urine and blood positive for glucose and ketones
    D. glucose in urine but not in blood

Questions 13-15.

DIRECTIONS: Questions 13 through 15 are to be answered on the basis of the following information.

Mrs. Eastwood, who is 65 years old, comes in with a complaint of painful swelling of the distal joint of her ring finger. A tentative diagnosis of rheumatoid arthritis is made.

13. Mrs. Eastwood is confused because her lab tests were negative, and she asks if she *really* has this arthritis.
 The BEST reply by the nurse would be:

 A. Don't think about it
 B. Eventually the tests will be positive
 C. Lab tests are often negative in the early stage
 D. None of the above

14. Mrs. Eastwood returns for the lab check and tells the nurse that she feels much better because she had been using aspirin, but she still feels a ringing in her ears.
 This may be due to

 A. the aging process
 B. cerumen in the ear
 C. involvement of the 8th cranial nerve because of aspirin
 D. otitis media

15. Mrs. Eastwood asks if she should take vitamins.
 The nurse's BEST response would be:

 A. Absolutely, they are good for you
 B. Older people need them badly
 C. There is no evidence that healthy older people require added vitamin supplements
 D. When you start vitamins, cut down on food

16. A patient with fatigue, shortness of breath, and swelling of hands has a history of rheumatic fever.
 On auscultation of this patient, you would expect the Si (first heart sound) to be LOUDEST at the

 A. right lateral border B. apex of the heart
 C. left lateral border D. base of the heart

17. When taking a history of a patient with glaucoma, the nurse should expect the complaint of

 A. seeing floating specks B. flashes of light
 C. loss of peripheral vision D. intolerance to light

18. The type of eye drop MOST commonly used in caring for a patient with glaucoma is

 A. pilocarpine B. atropine sulphate
 C. cyclopentolate D. tetracaine

Questions 19-23.

DIRECTIONS: Questions 19 through 23 are to be answered on the basis of the following information.

Susan, 47 years old, develops acute glomerulonephritis following a streptococcal infection.

19. During assessment, the nurse should expect Susan to report a history of 19.____

    A. recent weight loss
    B. mild headaches
    C. nocturia
    D. increased appetite

20. To prevent future attacks of glomerulonephritis, the nurse should instruct Susan to 20.____

    A. continue restrictions on fluid intake
    B. avoid physical activity
    C. seek treatment of any respiratory infection
    D. none of the above

21. Susan had extensive scarring and finally developed chronic renal failure. She is scheduled for a kidney transplant. 21.____
    After the transplant, the nurse should measure Susan's urinary output every

    A. 15 minutes
    B. 30 minutes
    C. hour
    D. 2 hours

22. The MOST important determinant that Susan's new kidney is functioning properly is 22.____

    A. white blood cell count
    B. serum creatinine
    C. renal scan
    D. 24 hour output

23. Signs of rejection of a transplant kidney include 23.____

    A. increased urine output
    B. elevated blood pressure
    C. weight loss
    D. subnormal temperature

Questions 24-25.

DIRECTIONS: Questions 24 and 25 are to be answered on the basis of the following information.

A 26-year-old college student is admitted to the hospital with a history of severe cramping and violent diarrhea of 2 days duration. A tentative diagnosis of salmonellosis is made.

24. Enteric precautions for salmonellosis include 24.____

    A. double bagging laundry
    B. wearing masks
    C. isolation
    D. limiting visiting hours

25. The diagnosis of salmonella is confirmed by 25.____

    A. CBC
    B. urinalysis
    C. febrile agglutinin test
    D. stool culture

KEY (CORRECT ANSWERS)

1. C
2. D
3. D
4. B
5. D

6. D
7. C
8. B
9. A
10. B

11. D
12. B
13. C
14. C
15. C

16. B
17. C
18. A
19. B
20. C

21. C
22. B
23. B
24. A
25. D

EXAMINATION SECTION
TEST 1

DIRECTIONS: Each question or incomplete statement is followed by several suggested answers or completions. Select the one that BEST answers the question or completes the statement. *PRINT THE LETTER OF THE CORRECT ANSWER IN THE SPACE AT THE RIGHT.*

Questions 1-6.

DIRECTIONS: Questions 1 through 6 are to be answered on the basis of the following information.

Mrs. Miller is 38 years old. She comes to the emergency room with the complaint of severe right upper quadrant pain. The pain started at midnight, when she and her family got home after attending a wedding.

1. At this point, you should include all of the following in differential diagnosis EXCEPT
   A. cholecystitis
   B. cholelithiasis
   C. ascending cholangitis
   D. acute peptic ulcer disease

2. Mrs. Miller states that she experiences mild pain off and on, mostly associated with fatty foods.
   The MOST likely diagnosis is
   A. ascending cholangitis   B. cholecystitis
   C. hepatitis   D. peptic ulcer disease

3. A diagnosis of cholecystitis with cholelithiasis is made. All of the following signs and symptoms may be associated with this diagnosis EXCEPT
   A. epigastric or right upper quadrant pain
   B. intolerance for fatty foods
   C. constipation
   D. pruritis

4. It is NOT true regarding cholelithiasis that
   A. it mostly occurs in women after age 40
   B. it occurs often in women taking oral contraceptives
   C. Caucasians and native americans are more commonly affected
   D. surgery is the only mode of therapy

5. The MOST common type of stones in cholelithiasis is
   A. calcium oxalate   B. calcium phosphate
   C. cholesterol   D. natrium acetate

6. The BEST way to provide nursing care to Mrs. Miller would be to
   A. administer pain medication and monitor for effects
   B. administer IV fluid as ordered
   C. provide small, frequent, lowfat meals if oral intake is allowed
   D. all of the above

Questions 7-12.

DIRECTIONS: Questions 7 through 12 are to be answered on the basis of the following information.

Mr. Sherwin is 28 years old. He comes to the emergency room with his girlfriend. He complains of severe diarrhea and abdominal pain. Crohn's disease had been diagnosed in the past, and he is experiencing an exacerbation.

7. Which of the following is TRUE of Crohn's disease?

    A. Mostly rectosigraoid area is affected
    B. Affects all bowel wall layers
    C. Diarrhea is almost always bloody
    D. Most commonly associated with colonic cancer

8. Dietary management of Mr. Sherwin's problem would include all of the following EXCEPT a high _____ diet.

    A. residue   B. vitamin   C. protein   D. calorie

9. Mr. Sherwin's problem would probably NOT be treated with

    A. antimicrobials   B. corticosteroids
    C. cholinergics   D. antidiarrheal

10. One of the nursing interventions for a patient with Crohn's disease is to provide appropriate nutrition while reducing bowel motility,
    This could be achieved by

    A. administering total parenteral nutrition
    B. providing a high calorie, high protein, low residue diet with no milk products
    C. administering antidiarrheals, antispasmodics, and anticholinergics as ordered
    D. all of the above

11. To provide or promote comfort and rest to a patient who is in the hospital with Crohn's disease, a nurse should do all of the following EXCEPT

    A. give narcotic analgesics
    B. provide sitz baths as needed
    C. apply protective ointment as needed
    D. provide good perineal care

12. The most important feature of Crohn's disease is that it can affect any portion of the gastrointestinal tract and, therefore, cannot be cured by surgery.
    Surgery is reserved for complications, such as

    A. fistulas   B. obstruction
    C. abscesses   D. all of the above

Questions 13-19.

DIRECTIONS: Questions 13 through 19 are to be answered on the basis of the following information.

Mr. Rosen, age 42 years, is admitted to the hospital with intermittent lower left quadrant pain. A diagnosis of diverticulosis is made.

13. All of the following are true of diverticulosis EXCEPT

    A. incidence increases with age
    B. most diverticulae are asymptomatic
    C. high fiber diet may be the cause
    D. occurs more frequently in developed nations

14. At midnight, Mr. Rosen developed a fever of 101°F and left lower quadrant pain. The MOST likely diagnosis now is

    A. peptic ulcer disease   B. pneumonia
    C. pancreatitis   D. diverticulitis

15. What would you expect on Mr. Rosen's lab tests after the fever episode?

    A. Leukocytosis and right shift
    B. Leukocytosis and left shift
    C. Leukopenia
    D. Eosinophilia

16. The MOST important treatment regimen at this point is

    A. high protein diet   B. IV antibiotics
    C. low residue diet   D. low fiber diet

17. Mr. Rosen's acute condition improved after appropriate treatment. Now, the mainstay of management should be

    A. high residue diet   B. laxatives
    C. stool softeners   D. anticholinergics

18. Nursing interventions for Mr. Rosen's diagnostic condition should include

    A. administering medications as ordered
    B. emphasizing the importance of adhering to the dietary regimen
    C. providing nursing care for the patient with bowel surgery
    D. all of the above

19. Surgical treatment would be warranted if Mr. Rosen showed

    A. repeated episodes of diverticulitis
    B. poor response to full medical and dietary therapy
    C. obstruction, perforation, or abscess formation
    D. all of the above

Questions 20-25.

DIRECTIONS: Questions 20 through 25 are to be answered on the basis of the following information.

Sonya is admitted to the hospital for surgical treatment of hemorrhoids.

20. All of the following are characteristics of hemorrhoids EXCEPT

    A. congestion and dilatation of the arteries of the rectum and anus
    B. bleeding with defecation
    C. pain with defecation, walking, or sitting
    D. may be internal or external

21. The procedure of choice for the diagnosis of internal hemorrhoids is a(n)

    A. barium enema B. proctoscopy
    C. endoscopy   D. digital exam

22. All of the following are predisposing conditions for hemorrhoids EXCEPT

    A. occupation requiring long periods of standing
    B. increased intraabdominal pressure caused by prolonged constipation
    C. hypertension (systemic)
    D. pregnancy

23. Sonya went to the operating room for a hemorrhoidectomy. Post-operative nursing interventions would include

    A. assessing for rectal bleeding
    B. providing routine post-operative care
    C. promoting comfort and elimination
    D. all of the above

24. Patient teaching and discharge planning for Sonya would NOT include information regarding

    A. dietary modification
    B. need to defecate when urge is felt
    C. avoiding use of stool softeners for first week post-operatively
    D. sitz bath after each bowel movement for at least 2 weeks after surgery

25. Sonya should be instructed about the recognition of and the immediate reporting to a physician of such symptoms as

    A. rectal bleeding
    B. continued pain on defecation
    C. pus-like drainage from rectal area
    D. all of the above

KEY (CORRECT ANSWERS)

1. C
2. B
3. C
4. D
5. C

6. D
7. B
8. A
9. C
10. D

11. A
12. D
13. C
14. D
15. B

16. B
17. A
18. D
19. D
20. A

21. B
22. C
23. D
24. C
25. D

TEST 2

DIRECTIONS: Each question or incomplete statement is followed by several suggested answers or completions. Select the one that BEST answers the question or completes the statement. *PRINT THE LETTER OF THE CORRECT ANSWER IN THE SPACE AT THE RIGHT.*

Questions 1-7.

DIRECTIONS: Questions 1 through 7 are to be answered on the basis of the following information.

A 42 year-old man is admitted to the hospital with fatigue, nausea, vomiting, weight loss, and liver enlargement. A diagnosis of cirrhosis of the liver is made.

1. Other signs and symptoms that you would expect with cirrhosis of the liver include 1.____

    A. irregular bowel habits
    B. increased abdominal girth
    C. changes in sensorium
    D. all of the above

2. Severe inflammation with massive necrosis as a complication of viral hepatitis would result in _____ cirrhosis. 2.____

    A. Laennec's
    B. postnecrotic
    C. cardiac
    D. biliary

3. This patient's _____ test would MOST likely be increased. 3.____

    A. serum albumin
    B. hemoglobin
    C. hematocrit
    D. prothrombin time

4. Which of the following tests would you expect to be DECREASED in this patient? 4.____

    A. Prothrombin time
    B. Serum albumin
    C. Serum bilirubin
    D. Alkaline phosphatase

5. A nurse can provide sufficient rest and comfort by 5.____

    A. providing bedrest with bathroom privileges
    B. encouraging use of soaps and detergents
    C. applying hot compresses to pruritic area
    D. providing warm and heavy clothing

6. Nursing interventions to institute measures to relieve pruritis include all of the following EXCEPT 6.____

    A. no use of soaps and detergents
    B. bath in tepid water followed by application of an emolient lotion
    C. apply hot moist compresses to pruritic areas
    D. keep nails short to avoid skin excoriation from scratching

7. Patient education and discharge planning for a cirrhotic patient would include all of the following guidelines EXCEPT:

   A. Avoid agents that may be hepatotoxic
   B. Avoid persons with upper respiratory tract infections
   C. May drink alcohol in a moderate quantity
   D. Self-assessment of weight gain and increased abdominal girth is important

Questions 8-13.

DIRECTIONS: Questions 8 through 13 are to be answered on the basis of the following information.

Mr. Davis, 45 years old, is admitted to the hospital with the complaint of painless hematuria off and on for the last 6 months. A diagnosis of renal cell carcinoma is made.

8. All of the following are characteristics of renal cell carcinoma EXCEPT

   A. most common site is bladder
   B. more frequent in women than in men
   C. peak incidence is from age 50-70 years
   D. medical management depends on the stage of the cell type

9. Predisposing factors to Mr. Davis' condition include

   A. chemicals, especially aniline dye
   B. cigarette smoking
   C. chronic bladder infections
   D. all of the above

10. Mr. Davis also has a history of recurrent urinary tract infections. While in the hospital, he complains about flank pain, urgency, frequency, and fever. You suspect cystitis. The BEST intervention would be to

    A. force fluids 3000 cc/day
    B. assess urine for odor, hematuria, and sediment
    C. administer antibiotics as ordered
    D. all of the above

11. The MOST common organism causing urinary tract infections is

    A. E. coli
    B. streptococcus pneumoniae
    C. staphylococcus aureus
    D. serratia

12. The treatment of choice for the organism MOST likely causing Mr. Davis' current problem is

    A. bactrim D5
    B. IV ampicillin
    C. ceclor
    D. nitrofurantoin

13. In patient teaching and discharge planning, to prevent urinary tract infections, Mr. Davis should be taught the importance of

    A. adequate hydration
    B. frequent voiding to avoid stagnation
    C. follow-up cultures
    D. all of the above

Questions 14-19.

DIRECTIONS: Questions 14 through 19 are to be answered on the basis of the following information.

Jonathan, who is 52 years old, is admitted to the hospital with severe right flank pain and bloody urine, but no fever.

14. What is the MOST likely diagnosis? 14.____

    A. Renal cell carcinoma   B. Nephrolithiasis
    C. Cystitis   D. Pyelonephritis

15. All of the following are predisposing factors to the diagnosis of nephrolithiasis EXCEPT 15.____

    A. diet containing large amount of calcium and oxalate
    B. increased uric acid level
    C. hypoparathyroidism
    D. sedentary lifestyle, immobility

16. Nursing interventions in a patient with a renal stone would NOT require 16.____

    A. straining all urine through gauze to detect stones and crush all clots
    B. forcing fluids 3000-4000 cc a day
    C. encouraging bedrest
    D. monitoring I and O

17. Jonathan passed a stone after 4 hours. It is found to be a calcium stone. Regarding Jonathan's diet, you should recommend that he 17.____

    A. avoid tea and chocolate
    B. avoid rhubarb and spinach
    C. limit milk and dairy products
    D. reduce foods high in purine

18. You should emphasize all of the following in Jonathan's teaching and discharge planning EXCEPT 18.____

    A. need for routine urine cultures
    B. need for routine urinalysis
    C. adherence to prescribed diet
    D. prevention of urinary stasis by maintaining increased fluid intake, especially in hot weather and during illness

19. Signs and symptoms of pyelonephritis include 19.____

    A. fever and chills   B. nausea and vomiting
    C. severe flank pain   D. all of the above

Questions 20-25.

DIRECTIONS: Questions 20 through 25 are to be answered on the basis of the following information.

Mr. Stevens is admitted for hemodialysis for renal failure. He has an external AV shunt.

20. To take care of an external AV shunt, it is important to do all of the following EXCEPT   20.____

   A. auscultate for a bruit and palpate for a thrill to ensure patency
   B. assess for clotting
   C. change sterile dressing over shunt weekly
   D. avoid performing venipuncture on the shunt arm

21. Around 11:00 P.M., you check Mr. Stevens' AV shunt and you notice that there is no pulsation in the tubing and the color of the blood is dark.   21.____
   The problem is PROBABLY that the

   A. arterial cannula is out
   B. venous cannula is out
   C. blood is clotted in the tubing
   D. patient has passed away

22. In the nursing care plan before and during hemodialysis, you should   22.____

   A. have the patient void
   B. withhold antihypertensive, sedative, and vasodilator medications
   C. monitor closely for signs of bleeding since blood has been heparinized for the procedure
   D. all of the above

23. Post-dialysis, Mr. Stevens is complaining of nausea and vomiting. You are worried that he has developed dialysis disequilibrium syndrome.   23.____
   You should look for all of the following EXCEPT

   A. disorientation   B. hypotension
   C. leg cramps   D. peripheral paresthesias

24. You should avoid all of the following on the shunt arm EXCEPT   24.____

   A. venipuncture
   B. skin care
   C. taking blood pressure with a cuff
   D. administering IV infusions

25. While the patient is having peritoneal dialysis, after the first few exchanges the normal dialysate outflow should look   25.____

   A. bloody   B. brownish
   C. cloudy   D. clear or pale yellow

KEY (CORRECT ANSWERS)

1. D
2. B
3. D
4. B
5. A

6. C
7. C
8. B
9. D
10. D

11. A
12. B
13. D
14. B
15. C

16. C
17. C
18. A
19. D
20. C

21. C
22. D
23. B
24. B
25. D

EXAMINATION SECTION
TEST 1

DIRECTIONS: Each question or incomplete statement is followed by several suggested answers or completions. Select the one that BEST answers the question or completes the statement. *PRINT THE LETTER OF THE CORRECT ANSWER IN THE SPACE AT THE RIGHT.*

Questions 1-8.

DIRECTIONS: Questions 1 through 8 are to be answered on the basis of the following information

Mr. Logmarino, age 55, has been a known alcoholic for the last ten years. He was brought to the emergency room because of confusion and hemoptysis.

1. All of the following are possible diagnoses of Mr. Logmarino's condition EXCEPT

    A. cirrhosis of liver
    B. ascites
    C. tuberculosis
    D. esophageal varices

2. Physical examination of Mr. Logmarino is LEAST likely to reveal

    A. peripheral edema
    B. shortness of breath
    C. hypotension
    D. changes in mental status

3. Mr. Logmarino's blood test would NOT show an abnormal increase in

    A. prothrombin time
    B. potassium (serum)
    C. sodium (serum)
    D. blood urea nitrogen

4. How would you modify Mr. Logmarino's diet to provide adequate nutrition to him?

    A. Restrict sodium to 200-500 mg a day
    B. Restrict fluids to 1000-1500 cc a day
    C. Promote high-calorie foods and snacks
    D. All of the above

5. The MOST important measure to take to prevent edema in Mr. Logmarino is to

    A. administer diuretics
    B. restrict sodium intake
    C. administer albumin
    D. measure input and output

6. After careful diagnostic tests and physical examination, the diagnosis of cirrhosis of the liver, ascites, and esophageal varices is made.
   If Mr. Logmarino begins to experience gastrointestinal bleeding, your PRIORITY should be to

    A. monitor vital signs more frequently
    B. administer fluid and blood
    C. inform the physician
    D. call the operating room for an emergency procedure

7. Mr. Logmarino had a Sengstaken-Blakemore tube inserted in an attempt to stop the bleeding. All of a sudden, he complains about respiratory difficulty. You should

    A. remove the tube immediately
    B. deflate the balloon
    C. deflate the balloon and oxygenate him
    D. remove the tube and re-intubate

8. Appropriate action was taken and the problem was discovered to have occurred due to tube dislodgement. To prevent this problem from reoccurring, you should put the patient in the _____ position.

    A. supine
    B. prone
    C. upright
    D. semi-Fowler's

9. The projections of renal tissue located at the tips of the renal pyramids are known as

    A. calices   B. papillae   C. cortex   D. medullae

10. A normal adult produces _____ of urine per day.

    A. 2 liters
    B. 500 cc
    C. 1 liter
    D. 5 liters

11. Which of the following parts of the renal tubule reabsorbs 80% of electrolytes and H_2O, all glucose, amino acids, and bicarbonate?

    A. Proximal convoluted tubule
    B. Distal convoluted tubule
    C. Loop of Henle
    D. Collecting ducts

12. The medical history, for assessment of the genitourinary system, should include any history of

    A. hypertension
    B. diabetes
    C. connective tissue diseases
    D. all of the above

13. Nursing diagnoses for the patient with a disorder of the genitourinary system may include all of the following EXCEPT

    A. sexual dysfunction
    B. alteration in comfort and fluid volume
    C. hematemesis
    D. alteration in thought processes

Questions 14-25.

DIRECTIONS: Questions 14 through 25 are to be answered on the basis of the following information.

Mr. Jackson, 55 years old, is admitted to the hospital with nausea, vomiting, diarrhea or constipation off and on, and decreased urine output. Chronic renal failure is diagnosed.

14. All of the following are predisposing factors to chronic renal failure EXCEPT 14.____

    A. recurrent infections
    B. exacerbations of nephritis
    C. hypertension
    D. smoking

15. Diagnostic tests of Mr. Jackson's urine would be LEAST likely to show elevated 15.____

    A. protein   B. calcium
    C. sodium   D. white blood cells

16. _____ would MOST likely be decreased in Mr. Jackson's urine. 16.____

    A. Specific gravity   B. Sodium
    C. Protein   D. White blood cells

17. Pre-renal causes of renal failure include all of the following EXCEPT 17.____

    A. decreased renal perfusion
    B. volume expansion
    C. congestive heart failure
    D. altered renal hemodynamics

18. Important nursing interventions in preventing neurologic complications in patients with chronic renal failure include monitoring 18.____

    A. every hour for signs of uremia
    B. for changes in mental functioning
    C. serum electrolytes, BUN, and creatinine as ordered
    D. all of the above

19. All of the following are signs and symptoms of uremia EXCEPT 19.____

    A. loss of appetite   B. confusion
    C. apathy   D. hypotension

20. Nursing interventions for a patient with chronic renal failure should include 20.____

    A. preventing neurological complications
    B. promoting/maintaining minimal cardiovascular function
    C. monitoring/promoting alteration in fluid and electrolyte balance
    D. all of the above

21. To assess and maintain a patient's maximal cardiovascular function, it is IMPORTANT to 21.____

    A. monitor blood pressure and report significant changes
    B. auscultate for pericardial friction rib
    C. administer diuretics as ordered and monitor output
    D. all of the above

22. One of Mr. Jackson's kidneys is found to be polycystic, and a decision is made to remove the kidney, which is contributing to renal failure.
The preoperative care of Mr. Jackson should include all of the following EXCEPT

    A. ensuring adequate fluid intake
    B. advising patient to expect flank pain after surgery if retroperitoneal approach is used
    C. assessing electrolyte values and correcting any imbalances before surgery
    D. explaining that the patient will have a chest tube

23. Post-operative care of Mr. Jackson would NOT necessarily require

    A. assessing urine output every hour (should be 30-50 cc/hour)
    B. weighing twice a week
    C. administering analgesics as ordered
    D. encouraging early ambulation

24. Patient teaching and discharge planning for a patient with one remaining kidney should include advice regarding all of the following EXCEPT

    A. prevention of urinary stasis
    B. avoidance of activities that might cause trauma to the remaining kidney
    C. no lifting heavy objects for about 1 week
    D. need to report unexplained weight gain, decreased urine output, flank pain on unoperative site, and hematuria

25. In Mr. Jackson's condition, which of the following would be an indication for dialysis?

    A. Progressive metabolic encephalopathy
    B. Uncontrolled hyperkalemia
    C. Intractable fluid overload
    D. All of the above

KEY (CORRECT ANSWERS)

1. C
2. C
3. B
4. D
5. B

6. B
7. C
8. D
9. B
10. C

11. A
12. D
13. C
14. D
15. B

16. A
17. B
18. D
19. D
20. A

21. D
22. D
23. B
24. C
25. D

TEST 2

DIRECTIONS: Each question or incomplete statement is followed by several suggested answers or completions. Select the one that BEST answers the question or completes the statement. *PRINT THE LETTER OF THE CORRECT ANSWER IN THE SPACE AT THE RIGHT.*

1. Bones do all of the following EXCEPT

    A. provide support to skeletal framework
    B. assist in movement by acting as levers for muscles
    C. provide site for storage of calcium only
    D. protect vital organs and soft tissues

2. It is NOT true of synovial joints that

    A. they are freely moveable joints
    B. they have a joint cavity between the articulating bone surfaces
    C. a cartilagenous capsule encloses the joint
    D. the capsule is lined with a synovial membrane

Questions 3-7.

DIRECTIONS: Questions 3 through 7 are to be answered on the basis of the following information.

Mrs. Wilson, 45 years old, is admitted to the hospital with the diagnosis of severe rheumatoid arthritis.

3. Physical examination will PROBABLY reveal

    A. painful joints
    B. muscle weakness secondary to inactivity
    C. subcutaneous nodules
    D. all of the above

4. All of the following would be included among the diagnostic test results for Mrs. Wilson EXCEPT

    A. various stages of joint disease shown by x-rays
    B. anemia
    C. elevated FSR
    D. increased white blood cells

5. Nursing interventions for Mrs. Wilson should include all of the following EXCEPT

    A. assessing joints for pain, swelling, tenderness, and limitation of motion
    B. promoting maintenance of joint mobility and muscle strength
    C. giving antibiotics
    D. promoting comfort and relief and control of pain

6. To ensure bedrest, if ordered for acute exacerbations, you should

    A. maintain proper body alignment
    B. provide a soft mattress
    C. keep joints mainly in flexion, not extension
    D. all of the above

7. On the day of discharge, you should teach Mrs. Wilson about the 7._____

    A. use of prescribed medications and their side effects
    B. performance of range of motion, isometric, and prescribed exercises
    C. importance of maintaining a balance between activity and rest
    D. all of the above

Questions 8-10.

DIRECTIONS: Questions 8 through 10 are to be answered on the basis of the following information.

Mr. Jacobs is 55 years old and has osteoarthritis.

8. All of the following are characteristics of osteoarthritis EXCEPT 8._____

    A. chronic nonsystemic disorder of joints
    B. women affected more than men
    C. degeneration of articular cartilage
    D. incidence increases with age

9. Nursing interventions in a patient with osteoarthritis, to prevent further trauma to joints and relieve strain, should include all of the following EXCEPT 9._____

    A. encouraging rest periods throughout the day
    B. ensuring proper posture and body mechanics
    C. encouraging walking without a cane
    D. avoiding excessive weight bearing activities and continuous standing

10. You would NOT expect to find _____ upon physical examination of Mr. Jacobs. 10._____

    A. pain and stiffness of joints
    B. Osler's nodes
    C. Heberden's nodes
    D. decreased range of motion

Questions 11-16.

DIRECTIONS: Questions 11 through 16 are to be answered on the basis of the following information.

Mrs. Fox, 35 years old, has been diagnosed with systemic lupus erythematosus.

11. During physical examination, the nurse should expect to find 11._____

    A. butterfly rash over malar eminences
    B. alopecia
    C. oral ulcers
    D. all of the above

12. All of the following diagnostic tests may be POSITIVE in Mrs. Fox EXCEPT 12._____

    A. antinuclear antibody   B. C-reactive protein
    C. LE prep   D. anti-DNA antibodies

13. Hematologic abnormalities in Mrs. Fox are LEAST likely to include

    A. hemolytic anemia
    B. leukocytosis
    C. lymphopenia
    D. thrombocytopenia

14. The LEADING cause of death in patients with systemic lupus erythematosus is

    A. infection
    B. renal failure
    C. skin disease
    D. CNS problems

15. Nursing interventions in this patient should include all of the following EXCEPT

    A. monitoring vital signs, I and O, and daily weights
    B. administering seizure medications as prophylaxis for CNS involvement
    C. assessing symptoms to determine systems involved
    D. providing psychological support to patient and family

16. Patient teaching and discharge planning for Mrs. Fox should include information concerning the

    A. disease process and relationship to symptoms
    B. need to avoid physical and emotional stress
    C. need to avoid exposure to persons with infections
    D. all of the above

17. All of the following would be included in nursing intervention for a patient admitted to the hospital with a fractured femur EXCEPT

    A. monitoring for disorientation and confusion
    B. performing neurovascular checks to the affected extremity
    C. avoiding analgesics
    D. encouraging use of trapeze to facilitate movement

18. In addition to routine care for a patient with open reduction and internal fixation, you should

    A. check dressings for bleeding, drainage, and infection
    B. turn the patient once every day
    C. turn to the operative side only
    D. all of the above

19. All of the following measures help prevent thrombus formation EXCEPT

    A. applying elastic stockings
    B. encouraging bedrest
    C. encouraging dorsiflexion of the foot
    D. administering anticoagulants as ordered

20. To prevent adduction of the affected limb and hip flexion in a patient with total hip replacement, you should advise the patient to

    A. cross legs
    B. avoid using a raised toilet seat
    C. avoid bending down to put on shoes or socks
    D. sit in low chairs

21. The *master gland* of the body is the _____ gland.   21.____

    A. adrenal   B. thyroid
    C. pituitary   D. parathyroid

22. The anterior lobe of the pituitary gland secretes all of the following hormones EXCEPT   22.____

    A. thyroid stimulating   B. antidiuretic
    C. adrenocorticotropic   D. follicular stimulating

23. Glucagon is secreted by _____ cells of the pancreas.   23.____

    A. alpha   B. beta   C. delta   D. gamma

24. A nurse would expect to find all of the following upon physical examination of a patient with Addison's disease EXCEPT   24.____

    A. muscle weakness
    B. bronze-like pigmentation of the skin
    C. hypertension
    D. weak pulse

25. Nursing interventions in patients with Addison's disease include   25.____

    A. administering hormone replacement therapy as ordered
    B. monitoring vital signs
    C. preventing exposure to infections
    D. all of the above

KEY (CORRECT ANSWERS)

1.	C	11.	D
2.	C	12.	B
3.	D	13.	B
4.	D	14.	A
5.	C	15.	B
6.	A	16.	D
7.	D	17.	C
8.	B	18.	A
9.	C	19.	B
10.	B	20.	C

21. C
22. B
23. A
24. C
25. D

EXAMINATION SECTION
TEST 1

DIRECTIONS: Each question or incomplete statement is followed by several suggested answers or completions. Select the one that BEST answers the question or completes the statement. PRINT THE LETTER OF THE CORRECT ANSWER IN THE SPACE AT THE RIGHT.

1. If the label on the bottle of sodium bicarbonate reads "0.32 gm. in 4cc," when the dosage ordered is grs, XV, you *should* give

    A. 0.15 gm   B. 0.20 gm   C. 0.44 gm   D. 0.96 gm

    1.____

2. In preparing to administer morphine, sulfate gr 1/8 (h) from tablets 0.010 gm, the accurate dosage would be _____ tablet.

    A. 1/3   B. 1/2   C. 3/4   D. 4/5

    2.____

3. If the label reads "Acetylsalicylic Acid 0.32 gm (grams)" for a 10-grain dosage, you should give _____ tablets.

    A. 2   B. 4   C. 5   D. 8

    3.____

4. According to Young's Rule, a child of 8 years will receive _____ of the adult dosage.

    A. 2/5   B. 1/3   C. 1/2   D. 4/5

    4.____

5. The dietary treatment of diabetes mellitus includes:

    A. Equalizing intake of proteins, carbohydrates, and fats
    B. Giving carbohydrates with restriction and adjusting intake of insulin
    C. Rigid restriction of carbohydrates and increased intake of fats
    D. Maintenance of body weight at optimal level

    5.____

6. In cardiac disease, the purpose of the low sodium diet is to

    A. relieve edema
    B. increase kidney function by changing the salt balance
    C. reduce weight through decrease of appetite
    D. make sure that the patient is salt free

    6.____

7. In fat-controlled diets,

    A. all fats are restricted
    B. fatty meats are restricted; dairy foods are unrestricted
    C. poly-unsaturated fats are substituted for saturated fats
    D. roast chicken is the preferred protein

    7.____

8. Of the following, the procedure which *violates* a law of physics and increases fatigue is:

    A. Working with the patient in center of bed
    B. Carrying a basin of water close to body
    C. Carrying a basin by placing palms flat around the sides
    D. Standing with feet apart

    8.____

9. The explanation of the fact that the comfort of the patient is related to the height of the headrest is: The _____ the headrest, the greater the _____.

   A. *higher*; distribution of body weight
   B. *lower*; distribution of body weight
   C. *lower*; strain on the sacrum
   D. *lower*; pressure on the buttocks

10. The "storage battery" which releases muscular energy instantly when a nerve impulse gives the order is a complex phosphate molecule commonly known as

    A. FAO   B. ATP   C. WHO   D. ITO

11. It is dangerous for a patient with a suspected malignancy of the gastro-intestinal tract to take sodium bicarbonate over an extended period of time because

    A. it hastens calcium metastasis
    B. its acidity is injurious to the tract lining
    C. it interferes with secretion of bile
    D. temporary relief pacifies the patient

12. The *approved* water temperature for the hot water bottle is:

    A. 105 degrees F - 115 degrees F
    B. 115 degrees F - 130 degrees F
    C. 120 degrees F - 150 degrees F
    D. 130 degrees F - 150 degrees F

13. Of the following items, the *one* that does NOT belong in the home medicine cabinet is

    A. an antiseptic   B. a lubricant
    C. a laxative   D. first-aid supplies

14. The value of the round-the-clock "q-4-h" temperature has been questioned because

    A. temperature has become less important in the treatment of disease
    B. it is known to vary with the time of day, month, age
    C. it is known to vary with individuals
    D. it wastes time of nursing personnel

15. Decubitus ulcers in bed-ridden patients are BEST avoided by the use of

    A. plasticized rings
    B. rubberized terry cotton draw sheets
    C. sheepskin
    D. polyurethane foam

16. The deciduous set of teeth does NOT contain

    A. cuspids   B. lateral incisors   C. bicuspids   D. canines

17. Adequate thermometer care is

    A. soap, water, friction   B. aqueous zephiran
    C. isoprophl alcohol 70%   D. alcohol 70%

18. The assimilation of calcium and phosphorus in the body depends upon the intake of vitamin

   A. A B. C C. D D. E

19. Gamma globulin is a protein blood fraction that carries antibodies. When injected, it provides

   A. acquired immunity
   B. active immunity
   C. passive immunity
   D. artificial immunity

20. On the centigrade scale, the reading of normal mouth temperature, 98.6° F, is

   A. 32° C B. 37° C C. 37.6° C D. 40° C

21. The oral (Sabin) vaccine against poliomyelitis contains

   A. inactivated polioviruses
   B. live attenuated polioviruses
   C. specific polio antibodies
   D. live monkey serum

22. Nursing care of the sick at home should be planned around the

   A. needs of the patient
   B. household routines
   C. economic status of the family
   D. needs of the family

23. Of the following, the vitamin that is NOT fat-soluble is

   A. A B. B C. E D. K

24. The SLOWEST of all sense organs to develop is

   A. taste B. smell C. sight D. hearing

25. The reaction upon which the tuberculin test is based is

   A. agglutination
   B. allergy
   C. antibody production
   D. precipitation

KEY (CORRECT ANSWERS)

1. D
2. D
3. C
4. A
5. D

6. A
7. C
8. A
9. B
10. B

11. D
12. B
13. C
14. A
15. D

16. C
17. A
18. C
19. C
20. B

21. B
22. A
23. B
24. C
25. B

TEST 2

DIRECTIONS: Each question or incomplete statement is followed by several suggested answers or completions. Select the one that BEST answers the question or completes the statement. PRINT THE LETTER OF THE CORRECT ANSWER IN THE SPACE AT THE RIGHT.

1. Radioactive carbon is a tracer element used to study the   1.____

    A. manufacture of erythrocytes
    B. motor nerve responses to stimuli
    C. path of certain food elements
    D. activity of certain endocrine glands

2. Mephenesin is used as a   2.____

    A. tranquillizer   B. respiratory stimulant
    C. muscle relaxant   D. respiratory depressant

3. Dextrostix are used as a one-minute test for sugar in the   3.____

    A. urine   B. spinal fluid
    C. gastric juice   D. blood

4. Cleft palate and hare lip have been developed in animals by depriving prospective animal mothers of certain vitamins during the period when the foetus' jaw and mouth are being formed. These vitamins are certain B vitamins and vitamin   4.____

    A. A   B. C   C. D   D. E

5. Edathamil calcium disodium may be administered before brain damage occurs in cases of diagnosed   5.____

    A. phenylketonuria   B. Wilson's disease
    C. lead poisoning   D. secondary anemia

6. Eggs contain an emulsifier of cholesterol known as   6.____

    A. lysine   B. lecithen   C. acetylcholine   D. trypsin

7. To ease the chronic shortage of high quality human bone available from bone bands, the Federal Drug Administration has approved the detailed processing of _____ bones.   7.____

    A. yearling lamb   B. six-months-old lamb
    C. six-weeks-old calves'   D. two-years-old cows'

8. The one-shot so-called "health gift" of measles vaccine contains _____ virus.   8.____

    A. dead measles   B. live measles
    C. mixed dead   D. mixed live

9. The diet prescribed for a phenylketonuria which may prevent brain damage is one that is   9.____

    A. *low* in fruits and vegetables, *high* in protein
    B. *high* in fruits, vegetables, and animal protein
    C. a commercially available protein substitute
    D. vegetables, fruits, and a commercially available protein substitute

10. The Haversian Canals are associated with the

    A. secretion of anterior pituitary gland
    B. aqueous humor in the eye
    C. excretion of pancreatic juice
    D. structure of long bones

11. A colles fracture is associated with the fracture of

    A. the lower third of the tibia - fibula
    B. the lower third of the radius
    C. a lumbar vertebra
    D. the upper third of the femur

12. In muscles undergoing contraction, irritability and fatigue may result from an accumulation of

    A. phosphoric acid
    B. carbon dioxide and lactic acid
    C. glycogen
    D. creatine

13. In the care of a patient who has suffered a cerebral vascular accident, the nurse's FIRST concern is

    A. rehabilitation of the patient
    B. helping to restore the confidence of the patient
    C. survival of the patient
    D. careful feeding

14. The procedure MOST frequently used to withdraw a small amount of spinal fluid for diagnosis is called a

    A. lumbar puncture
    B. cisternal puncture
    C. pneumoencephalogram
    D. ventriculogram

15. An infection of the kidney pelvis and the spread of the infection to the kidney tissue results in a condition known as

    A. hydronephrosis
    B. nephrosclerosis
    C. nephritis
    D. pyelonephritis

16. An *alternate* for insulin therapy in some cases of diabetes is therapy using

    A. sulfadiazine
    B. sulfaguanidine
    C. sulfapyrimidine
    D. sulfonylurea

17. When there is severe bleeding, it is usually best to IMMEDIATELY

    A. apply a sterile dressing
    B. apply a tourniquet
    C. apply a pressure bandage
    D. elevate the area

18. The PRIMARY function of protein in the body is to

    A. supply material for growth and repair of body tissues
    B. supply energy
    C. aid in the proper utilization of other nutrients
    D. transport vitamins and minerals to various parts of the body

19. *Good* diagnostic procedures used to give information about the heart are:

    A. Chest x-ray and electro-cardiogram
    B. Fluoroscopy and cardiac catheterization
    C. Lipiodal x-ray and B.M.R.
    D. Complete blood count and urinalysis

20. To avoid gastric irritation by frequent large doses of acetylsalicylic acid, the physician orders

    A. buffered tablets
    B. salicylic acid tablets
    C. aluminum hydroxide gel
    D. enteric coated tablets

21. The respiratory center is located in the

    A. medulla oblongata
    B. occipital lobe of the cerebrum
    C. corpus callosum
    D. cerebellum

22. The anatomical structure which performs the function of the nervous system is the

    A. neuroglia
    B. fibers of Remak
    C. neuron
    D. exteroceptors

23. Disruption of the erythrocyte membrane which leads to the cells' hemoglobin content going into solution in the plasma is known as

    A. agglutination
    B. phagocytosis
    C. hemolysis
    D. hemopoiesis

24. The cause of primary anemia is

    A. the inability of the patient to produce the erythrocyte maturation factor
    B. a poor nutritional pattern causing lack of hemoglobin
    C. sudden loss of large amounts of blood
    D. hereditary and may appear in any generation

25. Extensive superficial frostbite should be treated as deep frostbite, using a bacteriostatic agent and whirlpool bath of _____ water.

    A. cool   B. warm   C. hot   D. cold

KEY (CORRECT ANSWERS)

1. C
2. D
3. A
4. A
5. C

6. B
7. C
8. B
9. D
10. D

11. B
12. B
13. C
14. A
15. D

16. D
17. C
18. A
19. B
20. D

21. A
22. C
23. C
24. A
25. B

EXAMINATION SECTION
TEST 1

DIRECTIONS: Each question or incomplete statement is followed by several suggested answers or completions. Select the one that BEST answers the question or completes the statement. *PRINT THE LETTER OF THE CORRECT ANSWER IN THE SPACE AT THE RIGHT.*

1. The abbreviation *EEG* refers to a(n)

    A. examination of the eyes and ears
    B. inflammatory disease of the urinogenital tract
    C. disease of the esophageal structure
    D. examination of the brain

2. The complete destruction of all forms of living microorganisms is called

    A. decontamination   B. sterilization
    C. fumigation   D. germination

3. A rectal thermometer differs from other fever thermometers in that it has a

    A. longer stem   B. thinner stem
    C. stubby bulb at one end D. slender bulb at one end

4. The one of the following pieces of equipment which is USUALLY used together with a sphygmometer is a

    A. stethoscope   B. watch
    C. fever thermometer   D. hypodermic syringe

5. A curette is a

    A. healing drug   B. curved scalpel
    C. long hypodermic needle D. scraping instrument

6. The otoscope is used to examine the patient's

    A. eyes   B. ears   C. mouth   D. lungs

7. A catheter is used

    A. to close wounds
    B. for withdrawing fluid from a body cavity
    C. to remove cataracts
    D. as a cathartic

8. Of the following pieces of equipment, the one that is required for making a scratch test is a

    A. needle   B. scalpel   C. capillary tube   D. tourniquet

9. A hemostat is an instrument which is used to

    A. hold a sterile needle
    B. clamp off a blood vessel
    C. regulate the temperature of a sterilizer
    D. measure oxygen intake

10. Of the following medical supplies, the one that MUST be stored in a tightly sealed bottle is

    A. sodium fluoride
    B. alum
    C. oil of cloves
    D. aromatic spirits of ammonia

11. A person who has been exposed to an infectious disease is called

    A. a contact
    B. an incubator
    C. diseased
    D. infected

12. A myocardial infarct would occur in the

    A. heart   B. kidneys   C. lungs   D. spleen

13. The abbreviations *WBC* and *RBC* refer to the results of tests of the

    A. basal metabolism
    B. blood
    C. blood pressure
    D. bony structure

14. When a person's blood pressure is noted as 120/80, it means that his

    A. pulse blood pressure is 120
    B. pulse blood pressure is 80
    C. systolic blood pressure is 120
    D. systolic blood pressure is 80

15. The anatomical structure that contains the tonsils and adenoids is the

    A. pharynx   B. larynx   C. trachea   D. sinuses

16. An abscess can BEST be described as a

    A. loss of sensation
    B. painful tooth
    C. ruptured membrane
    D. localized formation of pus

17. Nephritis is a disease affecting the

    A. gall bladder
    B. larynx
    C. kidney
    D. large intestine

18. Hemoglobin is contained in the

    A. white blood cells
    B. lymph fluids
    C. platelets
    D. red blood cells

19. Bile is a body fluid that is MOST directly concerned with

    A. digestion
    B. excretion
    C. reproduction
    D. metabolism

20. Of the following bones, the one which is located BELOW the waist is the

    A. sternum   B. clavicle   C. tibia   D. humerus

21. The one of the following which is NOT part of the digestive canal is the 21.____

    A. esophagus   B. larynx   C. duodenum   D. colon

22. The thyroid and the pituitary are part of the _____ system. 22.____

    A. digestive   B. endocrine
    C. respiratory   D. excretory

23. The one of the following which would be included in a *GU* examination is the 23.____

    A. rectum   B. trachea   C. kidneys   D. pancreas

24. Of the following, the one which would be included in the x-ray examination known as a *GI series* is the 24.____

    A. colon   B. skull   C. lungs   D. uterus

25. A person who, while not ill himself, may transmit a disease to another person is known as a(n) 25.____

    A. breeder   B. incubator
    C. carrier   D. inhibitor

KEY (CORRECT ANSWERS)

1. D
2. C
3. C
4. A
5. D

6. B
7. B
8. A
9. B
10. D

11. A
12. A
13. B
14. C
15. A

16. D
17. C
18. D
19. A
20. C

21. B
22. B
23. C
24. A
25. C

TEST 2

DIRECTIONS: Each question or incomplete statement is followed by several suggested answers or completions. Select the one that BEST answers the question or completes the statement. *PRINT THE LETTER OF THE CORRECT ANSWER IN THE SPACE AT THE RIGHT.*

1. Thorough washing of the hands for two minutes with soap and warm water will leave the hands 1._____

    A. sterile
    B. aseptic
    C. decontaminated
    D. partially disinfected

2. The one of the following which is BEST for preparing the skin for an injection is 2._____

    A. green soap and water
    B. alcohol
    C. phenol
    D. formalin

3. A fever thermometer should be cleansed after use by washing it with 3._____

    A. soap and cool water
    B. warm water only
    C. soap and hot water
    D. running cold tap water

4. The FIRST step in cleaning an instrument which has fresh blood on it is to 4._____

    A. wash it in hot soapy water
    B. wash it under cool running water
    C. soak it in a boric acid bath
    D. soak it in 70% alcohol

5. If a contaminated nasal speculum cannot be sterilized immediately after use, then the BEST procedure to follow until sterilization is possible is to place it 5._____

    A. under a piece of dry *gauze*
    B. in warm water
    C. in alcohol
    D. in a green soap solution

6. A hypodermic needle should ALWAYS be checked to see whether it has a good sharp point 6._____

    A. when it is being washed
    B. when it is removed from the sterilizer
    C. just before it is sterilized
    D. immediately before an injection

7. Of the following, the LOWEST temperature at which cotton goods will be sterilized if placed in an autoclave for 30 minutes is 7._____

    A. 130° F   B. 170° F   C. 200° F   D. 250° F

8. Of the following procedures, the one which is BEST for sterilizing an ear speculum which is contaminated with wax is to

   A. scrub it with cold soapy water, rinse in ether, and place in boiling water for 20 minutes
   B. soak it in warm water, scrub in cold soapy water, rinse with water, and autoclave at 275° F for 10 minutes
   C. wash it in alcohol, scrub in hot soapy water, rinse with water, and place in boiling water for 20 minutes
   D. wash it in 1% Lysol solution, rinse, and autoclave at 275° F for 15 minutes

9. Assume that clean water accidentally spilled on the outside of a package of cloth-wrapped hypodermic syringes which has been sterilized.
   Of the following, the BEST action to take is to

   A. leave the package to dry in a sunny, clean place
   B. sterilize the package again
   C. remove the wet cloth and wrap the package in a dry sterile cloth
   D. wipe off the package with a clean dry towel and later ask the nurse-in-charge what to do

10. Hypodermic needles should be sterilized by placing them in

    A. boiling water for 5 minutes
    B. an autoclave at 15 lbs. pressure for 15 minutes
    C. oil heated to 220° F for 10 minutes
    D. a 1:40 Lysol solution for 10 minutes

11. A cutting instrument should be sterilized by placing it in

    A. a chemical germicide
    B. an autoclave at 15 lbs. pressure for 20 minutes
    C. boiling water for 20 minutes
    D. a hot air oven at 320° F for 1 hour

12. A fever thermometer used by a patient who has tuberculosis should be washed and then placed in

    A. boiling water for 10 minutes
    B. a hot air oven for 20 minutes
    C. a 1:1000 solution of bichloride of mercury for one minute
    D. an autoclave at 15 lbs. pressure for 15 minutes

13. The MOST reliable method of sterilizing a glass syringe is to place it in

    A. Zephiran chloride 1:1000 solution for 40 minutes
    B. oil heated to 250° F for 12 minutes
    C. boiling water for 20 minutes
    D. an autoclave at 15 lbs. pressure for 20 minutes

14. The insides of sterilizers should be cleaned daily with a mild abrasive PRIMARILY to

    A. remove scale
    B. prevent the growth of bacteria
    C. remove blood and other organic matter
    D. prevent acids from damaging the sterilizer

15. Of the following, the BEST reason for giving a patient a jar in which to bring a urine specimen on his next visit to the clinic is that the

    A. patient may not have a jar at home
    B. patient may bring the specimen in a jar which is too large
    C. patient may bring the specimen in a jar which has not been cleaned properly
    D. jar may be misplaced if it is not a jar in which urine specimens are usually collected

16. Of the following, the MOST important reason why you should remain with a 4-year-old child when his temperature is being taken by mouth is that otherwise the child might

    A. fall off the chair and fracture an arm or leg
    B. break the thermometer while it is in his mouth
    C. remove the thermometer from his mouth and misplace it
    D. leave the examining room and return to his mother

17. The BEST way to take the temperature of an infant is by

    A. feeling his forehead
    B. using an oral thermometer
    C. placing a thermometer under his armpit
    D. using a rectal thermometer

18. When the temperature of an adult is taken rectally, it is LEAST accurate to say that the

    A. temperature reading will be higher than if it were taken orally
    B. thermometer should be lubricated before use
    C. thermometer should be in place for at least ten minutes
    D. temperature reading is likely to be more accurate than if it were taken orally

19. When the temperature of an adult is taken orally, it is LEAST accurate to say that the

    A. thermometer should be washed with alcohol before it is used
    B. thermometer should be taken down below 96° F before it is used
    C. patient's temperature may be taken immediately after he has smoked a cigarette
    D. patient should be inactive just before his temperature is taken

20. The nurse described the test to the patient before bringing him to the examining room for a basal metabolism test. Her action may BEST be described as

    A. *correct;* the patient will be more cooperative if he knows what to expect
    B. *wrong;* the nurse does not know how the test will affect the patient
    C. *correct;* the nurse can judge whether the patient is too upset by this information to take the test
    D. *wrong;* explaining the test beforehand will only make the patient nervous

21. When a patient's sputum test is *positive,* it means that the 21.____
    A. patient's sputum is plentiful
    B. doctor has made an accurate diagnosis
    C. patient has recovered and is now in good health
    D. laboratory reports that the patient's sputum contains certain disease germs

22. A biopsy can BEST be described as a(n) 22.____
    A. pre-cancerous condition B. examination of tissues
    C. living organism D. germicidal solution

23. The *scratch* or *patch* test is USUALLY given when testing for 23.____
    A. allergies B. rheumatic fever
    C. blood poisoning D. diabetes

24. Gamma globulin is frequently given to children after exposure to and before the appearance of symptoms of 24.____
    A. measles B. smallpox
    C. tetanus D. chicken pox

25. Of the following, the one which is NOT a respiratory disease is 25.____
    A. bronchitis B. pneumonia
    C. nephritis D. croup

KEY (CORRECT ANSWERS)

1.	D	11.	A
2.	B	12.	C
3.	A	13.	D
4.	B	14.	A
5.	D	15.	C
6.	C	16.	B
7.	D	17.	D
8.	C	18.	C
9.	B	19.	C
10.	B	20.	A

21. D
22. B
23. A
24. A
25. C

TEST 3

DIRECTIONS: Each question or incomplete statement is followed by several suggested answers or completions. Select the one that BEST answers the question or completes the statement. *PRINT THE LETTER OF THE CORRECT ANSWER IN THE SPACE AT THE RIGHT.*

1. A physician who specializes in the treatment of conditions affecting the skin is known as a(n) 1.____
   - A. urologist
   - B. dermatologist
   - C. toxicologist
   - D. ophthalmologist

2. The branch of medicine which deals with diseases peculiar to women is 2.____
   - A. pathology
   - B. orthopedics
   - C. neurology
   - D. gynecology

3. The branch of medicine which deals with diseases of old age is called 3.____
   - A. pediatrics
   - B. geriatrics
   - C. serology
   - D. histology

4. *Petit mal* is a form of 4.____
   - A. epilepsy
   - B. syphilis
   - C. diabetes
   - D. malaria

5. Glaucoma is a disease of the 5.____
   - A. thyroid gland
   - B. liver
   - C. bladder
   - D. eye

6. A patient who has edema has 6.____
   - A. not enough red blood cells
   - B. too much water in the body tissues
   - C. blood in the urine
   - D. a swollen gland

7. The thoracic area of the body is located in the 7.____
   - A. abdomen
   - B. lower back
   - C. chest
   - D. neck

8. An electrocardiograph is MOST usually used in the examination of the 8.____
   - A. brain
   - B. heart
   - C. kidney
   - D. gall bladder

9. The word *coagulate* means MOST NEARLY to 9.____
   - A. bleed excessively
   - B. break up
   - C. work together
   - D. form a clot

10. A stethoscope is used to examine the patient's 10.____
    - A. heart
    - B. patellar reflex
    - C. blood cells
    - D. spinal fluid

11. A pelvimeter is MOST usually used in the examination of a patient in the _____ clinic. 11.____

   A. chest   B. cancer   C. prenatal   D. eye

12. Tuberculin may BEST be described as a 12.____

   A. virus infection of the lungs
   B. preparation used in the diagnosis of tuberculosis
   C. sanitarium for tuberculous patients
   D. form of cancer of the lung

13. An autoclave is a(n) 13.____

   A. automatic dispenser of instruments needed for clinic examinations
   B. sterile place for storing clinic supplies until they are needed
   C. apparatus for sterilizing equipment under steam pressure
   D. portable self-operating general anesthesia unit

14. Radiation therapy is 14.____

   A. the recording of electrical impulses of the body on a graph
   B. a study of the effects of radiation fall-out on the human body
   C. a form of treatment used for certain diseases
   D. the filming of internal parts of the body through the use of x-rays

15. Diathermy is the treatment of patients by 15.____

   A. scientific use of baths and mineral waters
   B. insertion of radium into diseased tissues
   C. intravenous feedings of vitamins and minerals
   D. electrical generation of heat in the body tissues

16. The measurement of blood pressure involves two readings, which are known as 16.____

   A. metabolic and diastolic
   B. systolic and diastolic
   C. metabolic and hyperbolic
   D. hyperbolic and systolic

17. The Snellen chart is used in examinations of the 17.____

   A. eyes   B. blood   C. urine   D. bile

18. An enema is MOST generally used to 18.____

   A. induce vomiting
   B. irrigate the stomach
   C. clear the bowels
   D. drain the urinary bladder

19. A bronchoscope is USUALLY used in examinations of the 19.____

   A. kidneys   B. heart   C. stomach   D. lungs

20. The Wassermann test is used to find out whether a patient has

    A. diphtheria
    B. leukemia
    C. scarlet fever
    D. syphilis

21. If a boiling water sterilizer is used, the minimum time necessary to sterilize instruments is MOST NEARLY _____ hour(s).

    A. 1/2
    B. 1
    C. 1 1/2
    D. 2

22. To sterilize towels and dry gauze dressings in the health clinic, it is MOST advisable to

    A. dip them in a sterilizing solution
    B. wash them with a strong detergent
    C. boil them in the sterilizer
    D. steam them under pressure

23. Sterilization by use of chemicals rather than by boiling water is indicated when the instrument

    A. is made of soft rubber
    B. has a sharp cutting edge
    C. has pus or blood on it
    D. was used more than 24 hours before sterilization

24. When dusting the furniture in the clinic, it is advisable to use a silicone-treated dustcloth CHIEFLY because the treated cloth will

    A. collect the dust more efficiently
    B. disinfect as well as dust the furniture
    C. not remove the wax from the furniture
    D. make it unnecessary to polish the furniture in the future

25. Assume that the clinic in which you work has issued instructions that all supplies containing poison are to have blue labels with the word *poison* clearly marked on the label, and that these supplies are to be kept in a storage cabinet separate from other supplies. You notice that a bottle with no label is on a shelf in the *poison* storage cabinet.
    Of the following, the BEST action for you to take is to

    A. place the unlabeled bottle in the back of the regular storage cabinet
    B. put a blue label on the bottle and write *poison* on the label
    C. ask another public health employee to help you decide if the bottle contains poison
    D. pour the contents of the bottle into the slop sink and destroy the bottle

KEY (CORRECT ANSWERS)

1. B
2. D
3. B
4. A
5. D

6. B
7. C
8. B
9. D
10. A

11. C
12. B
13. C
14. C
15. D

16. B
17. A
18. C
19. D
20. D

21. A
22. D
23. B
24. A
25. D

TEST 4

DIRECTIONS: Each question or incomplete statement is followed by several suggested answers or completions. Select the one that BEST answers the question or completes the statement. *PRINT THE LETTER OF THE CORRECT ANSWER IN THE SPACE AT THE RIGHT.*

1. When storing medical supplies, it is important to remember that liquids should be labeled   1.____

    A. only if the liquids are poisonous and there is the slightest chance that they will not be recognized
    B. whenever there is the slightest chance that they will not be recognized
    C. at all times and discarded if labels have become detached
    D. only in those cases where the liquids will be given to patients

2. When dusting metal counter tops in the clinic, it is BEST to use a clean cloth which is   2.____

    A. medicated   B. wet   C. dry   D. damp

3. Of the following statements concerning a hypodermic syringe, the one that is MOST correct is that a plunger   3.____

    A. used for taking blood specimens can be used with any syringe barrel
    B. can be used for any syringe barrel as long as it goes in easily
    C. can be used only with the syringe barrel that was made for it
    D. must be used with the syringe barrel that was made for it only if it is to be used for injections

4. The one of the following which should NOT be done when using a thermometer is to   4.____

    A. shake down the thermometer to 95° F before taking the patient's temperature
    B. ask the patient to keep his lips closed when taking the temperature orally
    C. wash the thermometer in hot soapy water after use
    D. keep the thermometer in a container of alcohol when not in use

5. The temperature of an adult when taken by rectum is USUALLY   5.____

    A. *higher* than if taken either by mouth or under the armpit
    B. *higher* than if taken by mouth and lower than if taken under the armpit
    C. *lower* than if taken either by mouth or under the armpit
    D. *lower* than if taken by mouth and higher than if taken under the armpit

6. Of the following tests, the one which is associated with tuberculosis is the _____ test.   6.____

    A. Schick   B. Mantoux   C. Dick   D. Kahn

7. A needle that has been used to draw blood should be rinsed immediately after use in   7.____

    A. a disinfectant solution   B. hot water
    C. cold water   D. hot, soapy water

8. Of the following, the statement that is MOST correct is that a hypodermic needle should be checked for burrs, hooks, and sharpness

   A. once a week
   B. before it is sterilized
   C. after it has been sterilized
   D. after it has been used three or four times

9. The MOST accurate of the following statements is that when a syringe and needle are being sterilized by boiling, the

   A. plunger must be completely out of the barrel
   B. needle should be left attached to the barrel as when in use
   C. plunger may be completely inside the barrel
   D. needle should be boiled at least twice as long as the syringe

10. Of the following, the MOST important reason for washing an instrument in hot, soapy water is to

    A. sterilize the instrument
    B. destroy germs by heat
    C. destroy germs by coagulation
    D. remove foreign matter and bacteria

11. Assume that a hypodermic needle which is to be used for injection is accidentally brushed at the tip by your hand. Of the following, the action which should be taken before this needle is used is that it be

    A. washed under the hot water tap
    B. wiped with a sterile piece of gauze
    C. washed in hot, soapy water, then rinsed in sterile water
    D. boiled for ten minutes

12. The CORRECT way to sterilize a scalpel is to

    A. place it in a chemical germicide
    B. boil it for 10 minutes
    C. put it in the autoclave
    D. pass it through a bright flame

13. Assume that a tray of instruments has been accidentally left uncovered for five minutes after it had been sterilized.
    Of the following, the action you should take to ensure that the instruments are sterile for use is to

    A. dip them in boiling water
    B. boil them for 10 minutes
    C. replace the cover on the tray
    D. wipe each instrument with sterile gauze

14. An intramuscular injection is MOST likely to be used in the administration of

    A. smallpox vaccine   B. streptomycin
    C. glucose   D. blood

15. The one of the following which is NOT a normal element of blood is 15.____

    A. hemoglobin B. a leucocyte
    C. marrow D. a platelet

16. Of the following statements regarding the Salk vaccine, the MOST accurate one is that it 16.____

    A. immunizes children and adults against paralytic poliomyelit is
    B. is a test to determine the presence of poliomyelitis virus in the blood
    C. is a test to determine whether a child is immune to poliomyelitis
    D. is used in the treatment of patients suffering from paralytic poliomyelitis

17. The GREATEST success in the treatment of cancer has been in cancer of the 17.____

    A. blood B. stomach C. liver D. skin

18. An autopsy is a(n) 18.____

    A. type of blood test
    B. examination of tissue removed from a living organism
    C. examination of a human body after death
    D. test to determine the acidity of body fluids

19. The word *vascular* is MOST closely associated with 19.____

    A. the circulatory system B. respiration
    C. digestion D. the nervous system

20. The word *diagnosis* means MOST NEARLY 20.____

    A. preparation of a diagram
    B. determination of an illness
    C. medical examination of a patient
    D. written prescription

21. A tendon connects 21.____

    A. bone to bone B. muscle to bone
    C. muscle to muscle D. muscle to ligament

22. Blood takes on oxygen as it passes through the 22.____

    A. liver B. heart C. spleen D. lungs

23. The fatty substance in the blood which is deposited in the artery walls and which is believed to cause hardening of the arteries is called 23.____

    A. amino acid B. phenol
    C. cholesterol D. pectin

24. The digestive canal includes the 24.____

    A. stomach, small intestine, large intestine, and rectum
    B. stomach, larynx, large intestine, and rectum
    C. trachea, small intestine, large intestine, and rectum
    D. stomach, small intestine, large intestine, and abdominal cavity

25. When giving artificial respiration, it should be kept in mind that air is drawn into the lungs by the 25.____

    A. expansion of the chest cavity
    B. contraction of the chest cavity
    C. expansion of the lungs
    D. contraction of the lungs

KEY (CORRECT ANSWERS)

1.	C	11.	D
2.	D	12.	A
3.	C	13.	B
4.	C	14.	B
5.	A	15.	C
6.	B	16.	A
7.	C	17.	D
8.	B	18.	C
9.	A	19.	A
10.	D	20.	B

21. B
22. D
23. C
24. A
25. A

EXAMINATION SECTION
TEST 1

DIRECTIONS: Each question or incomplete statement is followed by several suggested answers or completions. Select the one that BEST answers the question or completes the statement. *PRINT THE LETTER OF THE CORRECT ANSWER IN THE SPACE AT THE RIGHT.*

1. For terminal disinfection of thermometers, soak them in a solution of   1.____
   - A. 90% alcohol
   - B. merthiolate
   - C. mercurochrome
   - D. boric acid

2. Pure ammonia solution is   2.____
   - A. alkaline
   - B. acid
   - C. neutral
   - D. saline

3. In a reducing diet, use high protein content because protein has   3.____
   - A. high satiety value
   - B. low calorie value
   - C. low specific dynamic action
   - D. easy availability

4. Dextro-maltose is valuable in infant formulae because it increases   4.____
   - A. homogenization
   - B. digestibility
   - C. palatability
   - D. carbohydrate content

5. The substances that are non-miscible are   5.____
   - A. linseed oil and lime water
   - B. soap and water
   - C. glycerin and alcohol
   - D. olive oil and acetic acid

6. The substance known as *ACTH* is a secretion of   6.____
   - A. adrenal cortex
   - B. thyroid
   - C. anterior pituitary
   - D. pancreas

7. The tissue in which infection spreads rapidly is   7.____
   - A. adipose
   - B. fibrous
   - C. areolar
   - D. reticular

8. Boiling in water for ten minutes will destroy   8.____
   - A. non-spore forming microbes
   - B. spore-forming microbes
   - C. spore-forming pathogens
   - D. pathogens

9. The PRINCIPAL way in which germs enter the body is through   9.____
   - A. skin breaks
   - B. sex organs
   - C. nose and mouth
   - D. eye or ear

10. Fluorination of community water is

    A. definitely unsafe
    B. still in early experimental stage
    C. safe beyond reasonable doubt
    D. harmless but of little value

11. Simple goiter may be caused by lack of

    A. calcium   B. phosphorus   C. iodine   D. sodium

12. MOST finger stains may be removed from wallpaper with

    A. benzene   B. soap and water
    C. art gum   D. heat and brown paper

13. The *dominating gland* or master gland of all the endocrine glands is the

    A. anterior lobe of the pituitary
    B. pineal body
    C. adrenal cortex
    D. spleen

14. The physiological stimulant for the respiratory center is

    A. oxygen   B. calcium ions
    C. carbon dioxide   D. lactic acid

15. The MINIMUM time in which dishes may be disinfected by boiling in water is _____ minutes.

    A. 15   B. 10   C. 5   D. 2

16. Dichloro-diphenyl-trichoroethane is used extensively because it

    A. retains residual effectiveness
    B. is non-toxic to handlers
    C. does not burn
    D. dissolves in water

17. For lumbar punctures, the needle is USUALLY introduced just _____ the _____ lumbar vertebra.

    A. above; first   B. below; last
    C. above; last   D. below; first

18. Antigens used to stimulate active immunity are called

    A. serums   B. vaccines
    C. inoculations   D. injections

19. The soft part of the tooth that is susceptible to decay is the

    A. pulp   B. dentine   C. crown   D. root

20. The unit used for measuring acuity of hearing is the

    A. otometer   B. decibel
    C. audiometer   D. auditory ossicle

21. A mustard plaster for an adult with a normal skin should have a mixture of mustard and flour, respectively, in the proportion of one to

    A. two	B. six	C. ten	D. twelve

22. In illness, the importance of sunshine lies CHIEFLY in the fact that it

    A. induces relaxation
    B. supplies vitamin D
    C. increases morale
    D. is a powerful disinfectant

23. The change of nutrients into protoplasm is

    A. anabolism	B. karyokinesis
    C. osmosis	D. catabolism

24. The effect of heat on the vasodilator is to

    A. stimulate	B. deteriorate
    C. stabilize	D. inhibit

25. Painful effects of arthritis may be caused by

    A. chilling winds
    B. toxins from a disease germ
    C. complications of an infectious disease
    D. air conditioning

KEY (CORRECT ANSWERS)

1. B
2. A
3. A
4. D
5. D

6. C
7. C
8. A
9. C
10. C

11. C
12. C
13. A
14. C
15. C

16. A
17. D
18. B
19. B
20. B

21. B
22. D
23. D
24. A
25. B

TEST 2

DIRECTIONS: Each question or incomplete statement is followed by several suggested answers or completions. Select the one that BEST answers the question or completes the statement. *PRINT THE LETTER OF THE CORRECT ANSWER IN THE SPACE AT THE RIGHT.*

1. In diabetes, the body is unable to utilize

    A. vitamins
    B. proteins
    C. fats
    D. carbohydrates

2. The NORMAL inspiration rate per minute for the healthy adult is

    A. 8-12　　B. 16-20　　C. 24-28　　D. 30-35

3. The outside leaves of salad greens are important because they

    A. make the salad crispy
    B. are larger
    C. have more color
    D. contain more vitamin A and iron

4. Rubber goods should be stored in a

    A. cool dry place
    B. tin container
    C. medicine cabinet
    D. warm, moist place

5. Caffeine and strychnine stimulate the

    A. brain and afferent nerves
    B. brain and spinal cord
    C. autonomic ganglia and efferent nerves
    D. hepatic and pulmonary nerves

6. To get the required amount of vitamin C, consume

    A. cole slaw
    B. cocoa
    C. apricots
    D. whole wheat bread

7. Hyperfunction of the islands of Langerhans may cause

    A. hypoliposis
    B. hemorrhage
    C. hypoglycemia
    D. hypostalic congestion

8. The purpose of insuring regular rate of respiration is to reduce the amount of

    A. water in the body
    B. blood passing through the aorta
    C. carbon dioxide in the blood
    D. iron in the red blood cells

9. In destruction of microbes, the effect of heat is to produce

    A. liquefaction
    B. asphyxiation
    C. coagulation
    D. precipitation

10. The substance which is NOT a constituent of normal urine is

    A. ammonia
    B. creatinine
    C. hippuric acid
    D. indican

11. The GREATEST production care is given to milk that is labeled

    A. pasteurized
    B. approved Grade A
    C. homogenized
    D. certified

12. Lipase converts _____ into _____ .

    A. fats; fatty acids
    B. fats; proteoses
    C. proteins; amino acids
    D. sugars; fructose

13. Salts affecting acidity or alkalinity of protoplasm have the effect of

    A. osmosis
    B. condensation
    C. reduction
    D. buffer action

14. Temperatures of 0° F affect microbes to

    A. stimulate mitosis
    B. check multiplication
    C. destroy them
    D. attenuate the cellular wall

15. Baking soda added during the cooking of green vegetables to brighten their color also acts to

    A. destroy vitamin content
    B. destroy texture effect
    C. improve vitamin content
    D. improve flavor

16. The loop of Henle is a structural component of the

    A. aorta   B. pulmones   C. brain   D. kidneys

17. Two potential killers in the home to which the public has been alerted by the Department of Health, Education and Welfare are

    A. octachloro and methoxypromazine
    B. wax on milk containers and chlordane
    C. strontium 90 and nitrogen oxides
    D. polyethylene and aminotriazole

18. The body activity that is controlled CHIEFLY by the autonomic nervous system is

    A. coughing
    B. peristalsis
    C. walking
    D. sneezing

19. The basal metabolism remains unchanged in a person with

    A. nephritis
    B. malaria
    C. leukemia
    D. exophthalmic goiter

20. Excess glucose is removed from the bloodstream by the

    A. gall bladder
    B. liver
    C. small intestine
    D. pancreas

21. After proteins are digested, they are absorbed as

    A. peptones
    B. fatty acids
    C. glycerol
    D. amino acids

22. The membrane which does NOT form part of the eyeball is the

    A. conjunctiva
    B. sclera
    C. choroid
    D. retina

23. The process which increases the vitamin D content of milk products is

    A. homogenization
    B. condensing
    C. evaporation
    D. irradiation

24. A GOOD source of amino acids is

    A. carbohydrate
    B. fat
    C. protein
    D. citrus foods

25. Ultra-violet rays harm the eyes by

    A. drying out mucous
    B. enlarging the pupil
    C. spotting the cornea
    D. destroying visual purple

KEY (CORRECT ANSWERS)

1. D		11. D	
2. B		12. A	
3. D		13. D	
4. A		14. B	
5. B		15. A	
6. A		16. D	
7. C		17. D	
8. C		18. B	
9. C		19. A	
10. D		20. B	

21. D
22. A
23. D
24. C
25. D

TEST 3

DIRECTIONS: Each question or incomplete statement is followed by several suggested answers or completions. Select the one that BEST answers the question or completes the statement. *PRINT THE LETTER OF THE CORRECT ANSWER IN THE SPACE AT THE RIGHT.*

1. The sclera and chorioid tissues are found in the

    A. ear   B. heart   C. eye   D. stomach

2. The mineral which maintains osmotic pressure in the human system is

    A. iron   B. potassium   C. magnesium   D. sodium

3. Dishes used by a patient with a communicable disease should be

    A. boiled for 5 minutes in soapy water
    B. boiled in a creosote solution
    C. washed in clear water at 180° F
    D. washed for 5 minutes in soapy hot water

4. The natural source of insulin is the

    A. liver
    B. thymus gland
    C. pineal gland
    D. pancreas

5. Contaminated equipment should be cleared of spore formers by

    A. soaking in strong acid
    B. refrigerating
    C. dessicating
    D. intermittent autoclaving

6. Excessive amounts of alcoholic beverages over a period of time

    A. hamper the production of gastric juices
    B. reduce nervous anxiety
    C. dilate the blood vessels
    D. increase mental alertness

7. The MOST harmful drug derived from opium is

    A. heroin   B. morphine   C. cocaine   D. codeine

8. Novocaine is derived from the

    A. coca plant
    B. poppy plant
    C. hemp plant
    D. ergot fungus

9. Nissl's granules are found in the

    A. kidney   B. heart   C. brain   D. lung

10. The food substance which when absorbed by the body is MOST likely to increase the colloidal osmotic pressure of the blood is

    A. carbohydrates
    B. fats
    C. glucoses
    D. proteins

11. An acid ash is yielded by body oxidation of

    A. meats
    B. citrus fruits
    C. potatoes
    D. cream

12. A precursor of vitamin A is

    A. ergosterol
    B. carotene
    C. lysine
    D. pyrodoxine

13. Cells in the body which devour harmful bacteria are known as

    A. anthracites
    B. erythrocytes
    C. phagocytes
    D. parasites

14. At present, antibiotics are recognized to be

    A. a factor in altering the natural germ balance in the body
    B. ineffective in developing toxic reactions
    C. ineffective in developing allergic reactions
    D. most desirable in fixed antibiotic combinations

15. The study of pathogenic organisms in relation to disease is the science of

    A. microbiology
    B. blocking therapy
    C. chemotherapy
    D. replacement therapy

16. Atoms of an element that differ in atomic weight are called

    A. molecules   B. neutrons   C. isotopes   D. particles

17. The danger of strontium 90 lies in the fact that it

    A. is absorbed and concentrated in bone tissue
    B. causes tumors in smooth muscles
    C. falls back and is absorbed by the soil near the explosion
    D. renders the atmosphere unfit for breathing

18. Heat destroys bacteria by

    A. enucleation
    B. coagulating protein
    C. hemolysis
    D. making the cell wall permeable

19. The organ MOST commonly affected by arteriosclerosis is the

    A. brain   B. lung   C. kidney   D. heart

20. Some carbohydrates are required in a diabetic diet in order that

    A. sugars may be avoided
    B. fats may be oxidized
    C. loss of weight may be prevented
    D. intestinal putrefaction may be reduced

21. Carbohydrates are stored in the liver in the form of 21.____

    A. maltose   B. glycogen   C. dextrose   D. glucose

22. Ptyalin initiates the digestion of 22.____

    A. sugars   B. fats   C. starches   D. proteins

23. The enzyme which functions ONLY in an acid medium is 23.____

    A. pepsin   B. amylopsin   C. ptyalin   D. trypsin

24. Sulphonamides 24.____

    A. prevent the growth of bacteria
    B. destroy bacteria
    C. attenuate bacteria
    D. increase body resistance to bacteria

25. The part of the brain that is associated with memory is the 25.____

    A. cerebellum   B. pons varolii
    C. medulla oblongata   D. cerebrum

KEY (CORRECT ANSWERS)

1.	C	11.	A
2.	D	12.	B
3.	A	13.	C
4.	D	14.	A
5.	D	15.	A
6.	A	16.	C
7.	A	17.	A
8.	A	18.	B
9.	C	19.	C
10.	D	20.	B

21. B
22. C
23. A
24. A
25. D

TEST 4

DIRECTIONS: Each question or incomplete statement is followed by several suggested answers or completions. Select the one that BEST answers the question or completes the statement. *PRINT THE LETTER OF THE CORRECT ANSWER IN THE SPACE AT THE RIGHT.*

1. The compound which is NOT a constituent of normal urine is 1.____

    A. ammonia
    B. creatinine
    C. hippuric acid
    D. indican

2. A water solution of ammonia is a(n) 2.____

    A. acid   B. basic salt   C. base   D. acid salt

3. The substances that are NOT miscible are 3.____

    A. olive oil and acetic acid
    B. glycerine and alcohol
    C. soap and water
    D. linseed oil and lime water

4. The downward pressure of the water in an enema can depend upon the 4.____

    A. speed of flow
    B. size of the tube opening
    C. quantity of fluid used
    D. the height of the surface of the water above the patient

5. A stimulant for the respiratory center is 5.____

    A. carbon dioxide
    B. ethyl chloride
    C. oxygen
    D. nitrous oxide

6. The parts of the nervous system stimulated by strychnine are the 6.____

    A. hepatic and renal nerves
    B. brain and spinal cord
    C. autonomic ganglia and sciatic nerves
    D. coronary and pulmonary nerves

7. Solutions are absorbed MORE rapidly when 7.____

    A. they are in concentrated form
    B. they are slightly diluted
    C. spread over a large surface
    D. spread over a limited area

8. The effect of below-freezing temperatures on microbes is to 8.____

    A. destroy the pathogens
    B. kill them
    C. stimulate sporification
    D. check growth and multiplication

9. Boiling an article in water for 10 minutes will destroy   9.____

    A. pathogens
    B. non-spore-forming microbes
    C. spore-forming microbes
    D. spore-forming pathogens

10. An inexpensive disinfectant is   10.____

    A. bichloride of mercury   B. potassium permanganate
    C. creosote   D. alcohol

11. Vitamin A is stored in the   11.____

    A. skeletal muscles   B. liver
    C. thyroid   D. brain

12. Swelling, heat, and redness occur in an inflamed area because the capillaries become   12.____

    A. constricted   B. dilated
    C. ruptured   D. fenestrated

13. Bone owes its hardness CHIEFLY to the mineral salt   13.____

    A. calcium phosphorus   B. potassium iodide
    C. sodium carbonate   D. stearic acid

14. The number of vertebrae of the spinal column of a human is   14.____

    A. 33   B. 42   C. 28   D. 21

15. Sebaceous glands   15.____

    A. aid digestion
    B. have ducts
    C. are attached to the muscles of the eye
    D. increase blood pressure

16. Mastoid is   16.____

    A. a woman who practices massage
    B. marasmus
    C. part of the temporal bone
    D. inflammation of the breast

17. Morphology is a study of   17.____

    A. form   B. trench mouth
    C. death   D. the fetus

18. The Rh factors are   18.____

    A. negative   B. positive
    C. negative and positive   D. none of the above

19. Fungus is a

    A. form of plant life
    B. division of a nucleus
    C. medication for inducing sleep
    D. vitamin deficiency

20. Pigmentation

    A. depends upon the hemoglobin
    B. reduces body heat
    C. protects tissues of the skin
    D. produces color

21. In respiration,

    A. expiration is slower than inspiration
    B. receptors of the skin respond
    C. the hypothalmus is expanded
    D. enzymes are rendered inert

22. The permanent teeth in human adults should number

    A. 27   B. 32   C. 26   D. 34

23. The brain

    A. is dependent upon glucose for its energy
    B. functions in the final destruction of the red blood cells
    C. appears biconcave, is elastic and pliable
    D. separates the high pressure system of the arterial tree from the lower pressure system of the venous tree

24. Taste buds are located on the tongue and

    A. on the soft palate
    B. at the Eustachian tube
    C. on posterior descending branch of the coronary
    D. in the atrium

25. Metabolism

    A. expresses the fact that nerve fibres give only one kind of reaction
    B. summarizes the activities each living cell must carry on
    C. possesses the properties of irritability and conductivity
    D. describes the membrane theory

KEY (CORRECT ANSWERS)

1.	D	11.	B
2.	C	12.	B
3.	A	13.	A
4.	D	14.	A
5.	A	15.	B
6.	B	16.	C
7.	C	17.	A
8.	D	18.	C
9.	B	19.	A
10.	C	20.	D

21. A
22. B
23. A
24. A
25. B

TEST 5

DIRECTIONS: Each question or incomplete statement is followed by several suggested answers or completions. Select the one that BEST answers the question or completes the statement. *PRINT THE LETTER OF THE CORRECT ANSWER IN THE SPACE AT THE RIGHT.*

1. The heat of the body is maintained by   1._____

   A. oxidation   B. vertigo   C. gravity   D. hyperpnea

2. All cells   2._____

   A. exist proximal to liquid environment
   B. secrete a hormone which helps maintain the normal calcium level of the blood
   C. differ in origin and function
   D. are cone-shaped

3. The heart rate   3._____

   A. varies in individuals
   B. increases from birth to old age
   C. increases during first hours of sleep
   D. decreases in hemorrhage

4. A neuron consists of   4._____

   A. fluid in the semicircular canals
   B. conjugated protein which yields globin and heme
   C. a cell body and processes
   D. a band of spectrum colors ranging from red to violet

5. The process of swallowing is called   5._____

   A. delactation   B. diastasis
   C. deglutition   D. emission

6. Histology   6._____

   A. dissolves essential constituents in water
   B. connects arterial and venous circulation
   C. describes microscopic structure
   D. reduces diseased structures

7. When water is added to dry mustard, the reaction is   7._____

   A. polymerization   B. hydrolysis
   C. dehydration   D. neutralization

8. The efficacy of saline cathartics depends upon the   8._____

   A. selective action
   B. osmotic pressure
   C. relaxation of smooth muscle
   D. retarding of peristalsis

9. The chemical which stimulates the respiratory center is 9.____

   A. oxygen B. carbon dioxide
   C. calcium D. nitrogen

10. Carbon dioxide and oxygen are exchanged in the air sacs by 10.____

    A. infusion B. diffusion
    C. reaction D. filtration

11. The absorption of water through the intestinal wall is by 11.____

    A. filtration B. osmosis
    C. infiltration D. fusion

12. Oils and water do not mix readily because of the difference in 12.____

    A. heat of fusion B. surface tension
    C. heat of sublimation D. freezing point

13. The lowering of the head when a person feels faint will increase the blood supply to the head by 13.____

    A. suction B. gravity
    C. siphonage D. centripetal force

14. The ventricles of the heart act like a 14.____

    A. lever B. pump C. siphon D. barometer

15. A rubber hot water bottle transfers heat to the skin CHIEFLY by 15.____

    A. conduction B. convection
    C. radiation D. oxidation

16. A clinical thermometer is a(n) 16.____

    A. thermograph B. maximum thermometer
    C. minimum thermometer D. absolute thermometer

17. To increase the solubility of boric acid powder in water, 17.____

    A. increase the temperature of the water
    B. add boric powder rapidly
    C. decrease the area of contact with water
    D. supersaturate the water

18. The CHIEF component of Monel metal equipment is 18.____

    A. nickel B. copper C. chromium D. silicon

19. The contractility of the heart CANNOT be maintained in the absence of 19.____

    A. nitrogen B. hydrogen C. sodium D. vitamin D

20. Prolonged diarrhea can result in acidosis, due to loss of 20.____

    A. salts B. glucose
    C. body heat D. carbon dioxide

21. The fulcrum of an extremity is at the

   A. joint   B. bone   C. cartilage   D. muscle

22. Measurements of aqueous solutions are made from the bottom of the meniscus because water is _____ glass.

   A. adhesive toward
   B. absorbed by
   C. diffused through
   D. cohesive toward

23. Chemical heating bottles which employ the use of sodium salts produce heat by

   A. crystallization
   B. ionization
   C. fermentation
   D. hydrogenation

24. A rubber sheet is uncomfortable because rubber

   A. promotes evaporation
   B. absorbs perspiration
   C. is a poor conductor of heat
   D. is porous

25. The solution which should be administered through a glass drinking tube is

   A. sodium borate
   B. magnesium sulfate
   C. ferrous sulfate
   D. calcium carbonate

KEY (CORRECT ANSWERS)

1. A
2. A
3. A
4. C
5. C
6. C
7. B
8. B
9. B
10. B
11. B
12. B
13. B
14. B
15. A
16. B
17. A
18. A
19. C
20. A
21. A
22. A
23. A
24. C
25. C

TEST 6

DIRECTIONS: Each question or incomplete statement is followed by several suggested answers or completions. Select the one that BEST answers the question or completes the statement. *PRINT THE LETTER OF THE CORRECT ANSWER IN THE SPACE AT THE RIGHT.*

1. A forceps is a _____ lever.   1._____

   A. first class   B. second class
   C. third class   D. bent

2. Hydrogen peroxide disinfects by   2._____

   A. rupturing the bacterial cell
   B. precipitating protein
   C. bacteriostasis
   D. liberating nascent oxygen

3. Hot drinks increase body heat CHIEFLY by   3._____

   A. convection   B. radiation
   C. evaporation   D. conduction

4. A GOOD solvent for removing adhesive markings from the skin is   4._____

   A. rubbing alcohol   B. liquor antisepticus
   C. zephiran   D. benzine

5. If a thermometer is broken in the mouth, the mercury will NOT be injurious because the   5._____
   mercury

   A. has been treated to prevent chemical change
   B. will vaporize rapidly
   C. absorbs heat from the mucous membranes
   D. is in the pure inert state

6. The effectiveness of oral Penicillin is limited due to the   6._____

   A. need for greater purification
   B. formation of an insoluble compound
   C. irregular absorption
   D. irritation of the mucous membrane

7. The action by which dentrifices clean the teeth is CHIEFLY   7._____

   A. chemical   B. bacteriological
   C. mechanical   D. thermal

8. A difference between gamma globulin and polio vaccine is gamma globulin contains   8._____

   A. attenuated organisms   B. antibodies
   C. dead virus   D. antigens

9. Pulverizing a pill before administration will increase the speed of action by

   A. changing its chemical composition
   B. decreasing its solubility
   C. decreasing the alkalinity of the stomach
   D. increasing the surface area of contact

10. The virus in polio vaccine is

    A. virulent   B. inactivated
    C. suspended   D. emulsified

11. Antibiotics may produce

    A. imbalance in normal bacterial flora
    B. injury to blood forming organs
    C. inhibition of motility of the stomach
    D. injury to red blood cells

12. The PRINCIPAL organic constituent of perspiration is

    A. stearic acid   B. lachrymal
    C. urea   D. oxalic acid

13. The bactericidal action of perspiration is dependent upon its

    A. turbidity   B. viscosity
    C. pH   D. color

14. A substance which is NOT found in normal urine is

    A. urea   B. chloride   C. creatinine   D. acetone

15. Many of the bacteria which enter the stomach with food are either inhibited or destroyed by the

    A. high concentration of hydrogen ions
    B. mucin and salts
    C. gastric lipase
    D. enterogastrone

16. The tendon of Achilles is attached to the

    A. scapula   B. femur   C. calcaneus   D. clavicle

17. The hyoid is the

    A. u-shaped bone in the neck between the mandible and upper part of the larynx
    B. first of the upper seven vertebra
    C. breast bone
    D. knee cap

18. The ulna is located at or near the 18.____
   A. second cervical vertebra
   B. elbow
   C. arch into which the lower teeth are set
   D. knee cap

19. To test urine for sugar content, the proportion of urine to Fehling's solution should be 19.____
   _____ cc. to 1 _____.
   A. 3; tablespoon   B. 1; teaspoon
   C. 3; teaspoon   D. 1; tablespoon

20. The substance which is NOT found in vitamin B complex is 20.____
   A. nicotinic acid   B. thiamine
   C. prothrombin   D. riboflavin

21. The fat soluble vitamins are 21.____
   A. A, D, E, C   B. vitamin B complex
   C. A, D, E, K   D. A, C, E, K

22. The contraction of the heart muscle is caused by 22.____
   A. the systolic and diastolic (contraction and relaxation) periods
   B. many toxins accumulated in the blood by exercise
   C. the proper functioning of other organs in the body
   D. its own nerve tissue stimulated by chemical action of salts in the blood

23. The difference between the systolic and diastolic blood pressure is known as pulse pressure which should equal _____ millimeters mercuric pressure. 23.____
   A. 80   B. 60   C. 40   D. 20

24. The normal sugar content of the blood is APPROXIMATELY one part sugar to 24.____
   A. one thousand parts blood
   B. five thousand parts blood
   C. ten thousand parts blood
   D. none of the above

25. The nucleus of body cells contains chromatin. This substance is concerned with 25.____
   A. the process of cell division by which new cells develop through the process of mitosis
   B. chemical changes in foods
   C. the continued health status of cells
   D. the physical basis of heredity

KEY (CORRECT ANSWERS)

1. C
2. D
3. D
4. D
5. D

6. C
7. C
8. B
9. D
10. C

11. A
12. C
13. C
14. D
15. A

16. C
17. A
18. B
19. B
20. D

21. D
22. D
23. D
24. B
25. D

TEST 7

DIRECTIONS: Each question or incomplete statement is followed by several suggested answers or completions. Select the one that BEST answers the question or completes the statement. *PRINT THE LETTER OF THE CORRECT ANSWER IN THE SPAE AT THE RIGHT.*

1. Salts which affect the acidity or alkalinity of the protoplasm are said to have a(n) _____ effect. 1.____

    A. osmotic
    B. buffer
    C. condensation
    D. reduction

2. The vitamin destroyed by heat in the presence of oxygen is 2.____

    A. G   B. G   C. A   D. B

3. It is difficult to destroy tubercle bacilli in the human body because of the 3.____

    A. ability of the bacilli to form spores
    B. resistance of the bacilli
    C. rapid multiplication of the bacilli
    D. bacilli in body locale

4. In diseases of the liver, the diet should be 4.____

    A. *high* in protein and *low* in carbohydrates
    B. *high* in fat and carbohydrates
    C. *low* in protein and fat and *high* in carbohydrates
    D. *high* in carbohydrates and *low* in protein

5. When sodium fluoride is combined with calcium, it USUALLY _____ formation. 5.____

    A. retards acid
    B. speeds acid
    C. retards alkali
    D. speeds alkali

6. The thermatron is used to take temperature of the 6.____

    A. incubator
    B. vaporizer
    C. sterilizer
    D. blood donor

7. The destruction of red blood cells by sporozoites frees toxins which produce 7.____

    A. erythroblastosis fetalis
    B. malarial syndromes
    C. pernicious anemia
    D. primary anemia

8. The drug which has been produced without using molds is 8.____

    A. streptomycin
    B. chloromycetin
    C. aureomycin
    D. penicillin

9. A shielded concentrated source for deep therapy is 9.____

    A. Cobalt 60   B. Radium   C. Polonium   D. Plutonium

10. For close work, the foot-candle illumination should be AT LEAST

    A. 30 B. 10 C. 15 D. 25

11. Louis Pasteur is known for his work on

    A. tuberculosis
    B. smallpox
    C. puerperal fever
    D. rabies prevention

12. Ultraviolet rays are enclosed in quartz tubes because the rays can be

    A. uncontrolled
    B. measured
    C. filtered
    D. concentrated

13. Carbohydrate metabolism is GREATLY influenced by the following vitamin:

    A. thiamin
    B. vitamin E
    C. ascorbic acid
    D. vitamin A

14. Vitamin C deficiency causes

    A. weakened capillary walls
    B. nightblindness
    C. an increase in ear infections
    D. photophobia

15. Plasma is about _____ protein.

    A. 7% B. 80% C. 20% D. 75%

16. Lysol and creolin are used in solutions for hands in the strength of _____ percent.

    A. 1/4 to 1/4 B. 1 to 2 C. 3 to 4 D. 5 to 10

17. For terminal disinfection of thermometers, soak them in a covered dish containing 70% alcohol for _____ hour(s).

    A. one half B. three C. six D. twelve

18. The element essential in the biological oxidation of sugar is

    A. phosphorus
    B. sodium
    C. potassium
    D. iron

19. The addition of sodium bicarbonate in cooking speeds up the destruction of vitamin

    A. B B. D C. A D. C

20. Lymph is found in all of the following places EXCEPT

    A. pleural cavity
    B. bursae
    C. cerebrospinal fluid
    D. in the diaphysis

21. The application of sodium fluoride solution to the teeth will

    A. not prevent dental caries
    B. cause more harm than benefit
    C. not halt tooth decay once it has started
    D. discolor the enamel

22. The microorganism which has more than one cell is

   A. yeast
   C. diatom
   B. mold
   D. malaria plasmodium

23. Red blood cells

   A. fight infection
   C. carry food and oxygen
   B. give color to the blood
   D. discard carbon dioxide

24. Antitoxins are

   A. attenuated organisms
   B. dead organisms
   C. sera containing antibodies
   D. bacillary toxins

25. Fraternal twins come from

   A. the union of one female and one male cell
   B. two separate female cells and two separate male cells
   C. one female cell and two male cells
   D. two female cells and one male cell

KEY (CORRECT ANSWERS)

1. B
2. B
3. D
4. A
5. A

6. D
7. B
8. B
9. A
10. C

11. D
12. C
13. C
14. A
15. A

16. B
17. D
18. A
19. A
20. D

21. C
22. B
23. C
24. C
25. B

MEDICAL SCIENCE

EXAMINATION SECTION
TEST 1

DIRECTIONS: Each question or incomplete statement is followed by several suggested answers or completions. Select the one that BEST answers the question or completes the statement. *PRINT THE LETTER OF THE CORRECT ANSWER IN THE SPACE AT THE RIGHT.*

1. The one of the following which is a kidney operation is a   1._____
   - A. gastrectomy
   - B. nephrectomy
   - C. lobectomy
   - D. craniotomy
   - E. hysterectomy

2. The one of the following which is the medical term for nearsightedness is   2._____
   - A. myopia
   - B. strabismus
   - C. hyperopia
   - D. nystagmus
   - E. astigmatism

3. A patient with a Koch infection has   3._____
   - A. gonorrhea
   - B. syphilis
   - C. cancer
   - D. diabetes
   - E. tuberculosis

4. The one of the following which is the PRIMARY purpose of the Wasserman test taken during pregnancy is to   4._____
   - A. prevent congenital symphilis
   - B. find active cases of gonorrhea
   - C. prevent infection of the husband
   - D. prevent syphilis of the central nervous system
   - E. prevent luetic heart disease

5. Diagnosing cancer in its early stages is important CHIEFLY because   5._____
   - A. family members may be tested for hereditary predisposition
   - B. chances of cure are greatest when treatment can begin early
   - C. medication to prevent spread can be prescribed
   - D. cancer can always be cured when treatment begins early
   - E. the patient can be better isolated from contact with others

6. A cholecystectomy involves the removal of the   6._____
   - A. thyroid
   - B. colon
   - C. liver
   - D. gall bladder
   - E. spleen

7. A child has just recovered from acute rheumatic fever which has mildly affected his heart. The one of the following which is of GREATEST importance to him as a prophylactic measure is that   7._____
   - A. his family be aware of the situation
   - B. he attend a special class at school
   - C. he have no stairs to climb
   - D. he be on complete bed rest
   - E. he take care to avoid colds

8. The one of the following conditions which is NOT mandatorily reportable to the Department of Health is

   A. smallpox
   B. cancer
   C. poliomyelitis
   D. syphilis
   E. tuberculosis

9. The one of the following which represents the GREATEST value of special classes for children with marked eye defects is that

   A. there is less mental competition with normal children
   B. Braille books are made available to them
   C. sight conservation is taught and practiced
   D. corrective eye exercises are emphasized
   E. they can adjust better in the group

10. The one of the following diseases for which a sedimentation rate test is of GREATEST value is

    A. hyperthyroidism
    B. rheumatic fever
    C. pneumonia
    D. toxemia
    E. diabetes

11. Syphilis is caused by an infection with

    A. spirochaeta pallida
    B. gram-negative diplocci
    C. tubercle bacilli
    D. streptococci
    E. staphlylocci

12. The one of the following tests which is a basis for, or a confirmation of, a diagnosis of diabetes is a

    A. complete blood count
    B. darkfield examination
    C. spinal fluid examination
    D. patch test
    E. glucose tolerance test

13. The one of the following diseases which is caused by a deficiency of vitamin D is

    A. rickets
    B. pellagra
    C. beriberi
    D. scurvy
    E. anemia

14. The one of the following diseases which has been MOST prevalent in the United States in the last five years is

    A. heart disease
    B. typhoid
    C. poliomyelitis
    D. tuberculosis
    E. cancer

15. In establishing a diagnosis of pulmonary tuberculosis, the one of the following which is MOST valuable to the doctor is

    A. the Mantoux test
    B. Roentgen study
    C. gastric lavago
    D. a thermometer
    E. fluoroscopic study

16. The one of the following which is the MOST common cause of death from heart disease in the age group of one week to five years is

    A. hypertension
    B. angina pectoris
    C. syphilitic heart disease
    D. congenital heart disease
    E. rheumatic heart disease

17. According to our present knowledge of the effects of certain diseases during the first three months of pregnancy, the one of the following diseases which would have the MOST harmful effect on the unborn fetus is

    A. German measles
    B. gonorrhea
    C. heart disease
    D. lobar pneumonia
    E. thrombophlebitis

18. According to the American Heart Association's classification, a 24-year-old female patient classified as Functional, Class IA would be

    A. on complete bed rest
    B. warned against pregnancies
    C. allowed normal activity
    D. on a convalescent status
    E. restrained from any stair climbing

19. The one of the following diseases which is caused by a birth injury is

    A. cerebral palsy
    B. meningitis
    C. hydrocele
    D. congenital syphilis
    E. epilepsy

20. In helping a patient who has arteriosclerotic heart disease to plan for his future, the one of the following phases on which you would specifically seek information from the patient's doctor is the

    A. emotional basis of the illness
    B. etiology of the disease process
    C. functioning capacity of the patient
    D. awareness of hereditary predisposition
    E. anatomical changes which have occurred

21. The one of the following eye conditions which is MOST commonly found in the premature infant is

    A. strabismus
    B. myopia
    C. phylctenular keratitis
    D. retrolental fibroplasia
    E. glaucoma

22. The one of the following cases in which eclampsia is MOST likely to occur is

    A. diabetes
    B. shock therapy
    C. syphilitic infection
    D. measles
    E. pregnancy

23. A delusion is a

    A. disharmony of mind and body
    B. fantastic image formed during sleep

C. false judgment of objective things
D. cessation of thought
E. distorted perception or image

24. The one of the following which is the MOST common form of treatment employed by psychiatrists in treating patients with mental disorders is

   A. hypnotism	B. hydrotherapy	C. electroshock
   D. insulin shock	E. psychotherapy

25. A masochistic person is one who

   A. is very melancholy
   B. has delusions of grandeur about himself
   C. derives pleasure from being cruelly treated
   D. believes in a fatalistic philosophy
   E. derives pleasure from hurting another

26. Surgery is ESPECIALLY difficult during the oedipal period because of the

   A. father attachment	B. mental age
   C. castration anxieties	D. rejection complex
   E. separation from siblings

27. A psychometric test is one which attempts to measure

   A. social adjustment	B. emotional maturity
   C. physical activity	D. personality development
   E. intellectual capacity

28. The one of the following conditions which falls into the classification of a psychosis rather than psychoneurosis is

   A. anxiety hysteria	B. schizophrenia
   C. neurasthenia	D. conversion hysteria
   E. compulsion neurosis

29. The one of the following which BEST describes psychosomatic medicine is

   A. the understanding and treatment of both mind and body in illness
   B. the treatment of disease by psychiatric methods only
   C. the separation of mind and body in medical treatment
   D. the psychological testing of all individuals
   E. a system of socialized medical planning

30. The one of the following conditions for which shock treatment is FREQUENTLY used is

   A. alcoholism	B. Parkinson's syndrome
   C. multiple sclerosis	D. schizophrenia
   E. diabetes

31. The incidence of any particular disease is called the _____ rate.

   A. mortality	B. morbidity	C. endemic
   D. death	E. differential

32. The one of the following which is the PRIMARY purpose of the mass chest x-ray surveys is to

    A. find active cases of tuberculosis
    B. give early treatment for tuberculosis
    C. educate the public
    D. lower the death rate among the aged
    E. carry out a research project

33. When a child develops whooping cough after having been closely exposed to the disease, the cause is said to be

    A. endogenous   B. exogenous   C. endemic
    D. endoglobular   E. ectatic

34. The one of the following diseases for which the necessary medication will be given free by the Department of Health is

    A. poliomyelitis   B. pneumonia   C. cancer
    D. syphilis   E. epilepsy

35. The branch of medical science which deals with the conditions of the older age group is called

    A. pediatrics   B. dietetics   C. gerontology
    D. orthopedics   E. cardiology

KEY (CORRECT ANSWERS)

1.	B	16.	D
2.	A	17.	A
3.	E	18.	C
4.	A	19.	A
5.	B	20.	C
6.	D	21.	D
7.	E	22.	E
8.	B	23.	C
9.	C	24.	E
10.	B	25.	C
11.	A	26.	C
12.	E	27.	E
13.	A	28.	B
14.	A	29.	A
15.	B	30.	D

31. B
32. A
33. B
34. D
35. C

TEST 2

DIRECTIONS: Each question or incomplete statement is followed by several suggested answers or completions. Select the one that BEST answers the question or completes the statement. *PRINT THE LETTER OF THE CORRECT ANSWER IN THE SPACE AT THE RIGHT.*

1. Eclampsia is MOST likely to occur in the course of

   A. pregnancy
   B. poliomyelitis
   C. German measles
   D. scarlet fever

   1.____

2. The one of the following diseases which is characterized by an overabundance of white cells in the body is

   A. hemophilia
   B. polycythemia
   C. anemia
   D. leucemia

   2.____

3. The GREATEST single factor in improving the prognosis in diabetes in children is

   A. improvement in standards of living
   B. the discovery of insulin
   C. greater emphasis on prenatal care
   D. improved surgical techniques

   3.____

4. The one of the following which FREQUENTLY causes a baby to be cyanotic at birth is

   A. a neurological disorder
   B. congenital heart disease
   C. gonorrhea
   D. tuberculosis

   4.____

5. In establishing a diagnosis of *grand mal*, the one of the following which would be MOST helpful to the doctor is an(the)

   A. electrocardiogram
   B. encephalogram
   C. basal metabolism rate
   D. blood pressure reading

   5.____

6. Oophorectomy is a surgical procedure involving removal of the

   A. kidney
   B. brain lobe
   C. ovary
   D. thyroid gland

   6.____

7. The one of the following laboratory procedures which is used SPECIFICALLY in diagnosing cancer is a

   A. glucose tolerance test
   B. dark-field examination
   C. blood test
   D. Papanicolaou smear

   7.____

8. Cerebral palsy is known as _____ disease.

   A. Pott's   B. Little's   C. Addison's   D. Grave's

   8.____

9. An electroencephalogram is used in establishing a diagnosis of

   A. rheumatic heart disease
   B. cholecystitis
   C. Hodgkin's disease
   D. epilepsy

   9.____

10. The one of the following conditions which is NOT caused by the dysfunction of endocrine glands is

   A. myxedema
   B. duodenal ulcer
   C. cretinism
   D. Addison's disease

11. A diagnostic procedure used in determining the presence of syphilis is a

   A. patch test
   B. dark-field examination
   C. sputum test
   D. gastric analysis

12. An eye condition necessitating the use of glasses which COMMONLY appears with the advent of middle age is

   A. myopia
   B. strabismus
   C. presbyopia
   D. fibroplasia

13. The one of the following laboratory tests which is performed to determine or confirm the presence of central nervous system syphilis is a

   A. glucose tolerance test
   B. sedimentation test
   C. colloidal gold test
   D. Papanicolaou smear

14. A COMMON surgical procedure used in the treatment of duodenal ulcer is

   A. nephrectomy
   B. cholecystectomy
   C. lobectomy
   D. subtotal gastrectomy

15. The one of the following tests which is used to determine the presence of dysfunction of the thyroid gland is

   A. a sputum test
   B. an electroencephalogram
   C. gastric analysis
   D. a basal metabolism test

16. The MOST effective antibiotic in present-day treatment of syphilis is

   A. penicillin
   B. streptomycin
   C. terramycin
   D. aureomycin

17. The one of the following which is COMMONLY used to determine the presence of a brain tumor is

   A. a cardiogram
   B. urinalysis
   C. a glucose tolerance test
   D. a ventriculogram

18. Under the Sanitary Code, it is necessary to report the positive results of certain tests or specimen examinations to the Department of Health within 24 hours.
    The one of the following which does NOT have to be reported is

   A. a positive Zondek-Aschheim test
   B. the presence of Klebs-Loeffler bacilli
   C. the presence of bacillus typhosus
   D. a positive Kline-Young test

19. A curette is a

   A. healing drug
   B. curved scalpel
   C. long hypodermic needle
   D. scraping instrument

20. A myocardial infarct would occur in the   20._____

   A. heart   B. kidneys   C. lungs   D. spleen

Questions 21-25.

DIRECTIONS: For Questions 21 through 25, Column I lists body organs and Column II lists names of surgical procedures. For each body organ listed in Column I, select the surgical procedure in Column II which involves the organ, and write the letter which precedes the surgical procedure in the answer blank corresponding to the number of the question.

COLUMN I   COLUMN II

21. Brain   A. Cholecystectomy   21._____
22. Gall bladder   B. Enucleation   22._____
23. Larynx   C. Gastrectomy   23._____
24. Reproductive organs D. Lobotomy   24._____
25. Stomach   E. Nephrectomy   25._____
                        F. Orchidectomy
                        G. Tracheotomy

KEY (CORRECT ANSWERS)

1. A   11. B
2. D   12. C
3. B   13. C
4. B   14. D
5. B   15. D

6. C   16. A
7. D   17. D
8. B   18. A
9. D   19. D
10. B   20. A

21. D
22. A
23. G
24. F
25. C

BASIC FUNDAMENTALS OF MEDICATION ADMINISTRATION

CONTENTS

	Page
I. GUIDELINES FOR MEDICATION ADMINISTRATION	1
A. General	1
B. Unit Dose	3
II. MEDICATION ADMINISTRATION RECORD	4
III. DROPS	7
A. Ear	7
B. Eye	8
C. Nose	9
IV. GASTRIC TUBES	10
V. HEPARIN LOCKS	11
VI. INJECTIONS	12
A. General	12
B. Intramuscular	14
1. Z-Tract	15
C. Intradermal	15
D. Intravenous Piggyback	16
E. Subcutaneous	18
1. Insulin	18
VII. ORAL MEDICATIONS	19
A. Tablets, Pills, or Capsules	20
B. Powders	20
C. Liquids	20
VIII. SUPPOSITORIES	21
A. Rectal	21
B. Urethral	22
C. Vaginal	23

BASIC FUNDAMENTALS OF MEDICATION ADMINISTRATION

I. GUIDELINES FOR MEDICATION ADMINISTRATION

A. General

PURPOSE

To administer the right medication, in the right dose, by the right route, to the right patient, at the right time

PROCEDURE	SPECIAL CONSIDERATIONS
• Transcribe medication and treatment orders from doctor's orders to • Medication and Treatment Cards • Nursing Care Plan • Medication Administration Record (MAR)	Follow local policy.
• Check ALL Medication and Treatment Cards against Nursing Care Plan at the beginning of each shift.	
• Return cards to medication and treatment board, placing each card in space corresponding to hour when medication is due. • Clean working area.	
• Wash your hands.	
• Obtain supplies and equipment such as tongue blades, paper cups, pitcher of water, medication tray or cart, and stethoscope.	Keep cards for same patient together.
• Separate cards into • oral medications • injections • treatments	
• Arrange cards in sequence similar to placement of patients on ward.	
• Turn cards face down, turn top card up, and read information on card.	
• Locate medication and compare label on medication with name of medication and dosage on card.	FIRST MEDICATION CHECK.

GUIDELINES FOR MEDICATION ADMINISTRATION, GENERAL (cont)

PROCEDURE	SPECIAL CONSIDERATIONS
• Remove medication container and compare label on container with name of medication and dosage on card.	SECOND CHECK.
• Pour required dosage and compare label on container with card for name of medication and dosage.	THIRD CHECK.
• Place medication and card on tray or cart.	NEVER leave medication cart or tray unattended.
• Continue with remaining cards in same manner.	
• Lock medication cabinet before leaving the area.	
• Administer only medications that you personally prepared.	NEVER allow others to administer medication that you prepared.
• Check name on bed tag with name on card.	FIRST ID CHECK.
• Compare name on card with patient's ID band.	SECOND CHECK.
• Ask patient: "What is your name?" Be sure response is accurate.	THIRD CHECK.
• Administer medication ONLY if all 3 checks agree.	
• Place card face down on one side of tray.	
• Continue to administer medications until all are given.	
• Reset tray or cart for next use.	
• Take cards to desk.	
• Record medications, time and date given, and your initials on MAR using cards as guide.	
• Replace cards on board at next hour due.	

B. *Unit Dose*

PURPOSE

To administer single-dose medication in ready-to-use form

PROCEDURE

- See "Guidelines for Medication Administration, General."

- Get stocked medication cart from storage area.

- Unlock cart.

- Wheel medication cart to bedside, check MAR, and identify patient.

- Open cassette drawer.
    - Read MAR.
    - Select medication from cassette drawer.

- Check medication against MAR for date, dosage, and route.

- Administer medication and record immediately on MAR.
    - Remain with patient until medication has been taken.
    - Replace drawer in correct space in cassette.

- Dispose of litter, syringe, and needle before moving to next patient.
    - Break off tip of needle and syringe, and dispose in dirty needle box.
    - Place glass unit dose liquid container in bag for return to pharmacy.

- Lock cart and return to storage area.

SPECIAL CONSIDERATIONS

Cart is stocked by pharmacy personnel.

Follow local policy.

II. MEDICATION ADMINISTRATION RECORD (MAR)

PURPOSE
To maintain a permanent record of medication administered

PROCEDURE	SPECIAL CONSIDERATIONS
•Stamp MAR with Addressograph as shown in figure 6-1 on the following page.	
• Enter ward number at bottom right of form; record month and year in space provided at the top.	Make all entries in black ink.
• Transcribe scheduled medications from doctor's orders to front of form.	
• Enter order date, medication dosage, frequency, and route of administration.	
• Complete "Hours" column to indicate scheduled hours for administration starting with earliest military time after 2400 hours.	
• Complete "Dates Given" blocks at top of form.	
• Enter month and dates for a 7day period, starting with first day medication is given.	
• Cancel vacant spaces with an "X."	
• Draw a heavy line across page under last entry and enter next medication directly below.	Do not skip a space.
• When medication has been given, enter your initials in column corresponding to date and hour of administration.	
• Place an "*" in column if the medication was .not given and state reason on Nursing Notes.	
• Place an "L" under date and opposite hour patient is on liberty.	Follow local policy.
• When medication is stopped, bracket remaining spaces for that day; write "STOPPED," enter date and initials.	Applies to scheduled drugs, PRN, and variable dose medications.
• Complete "Initial Code" section.	

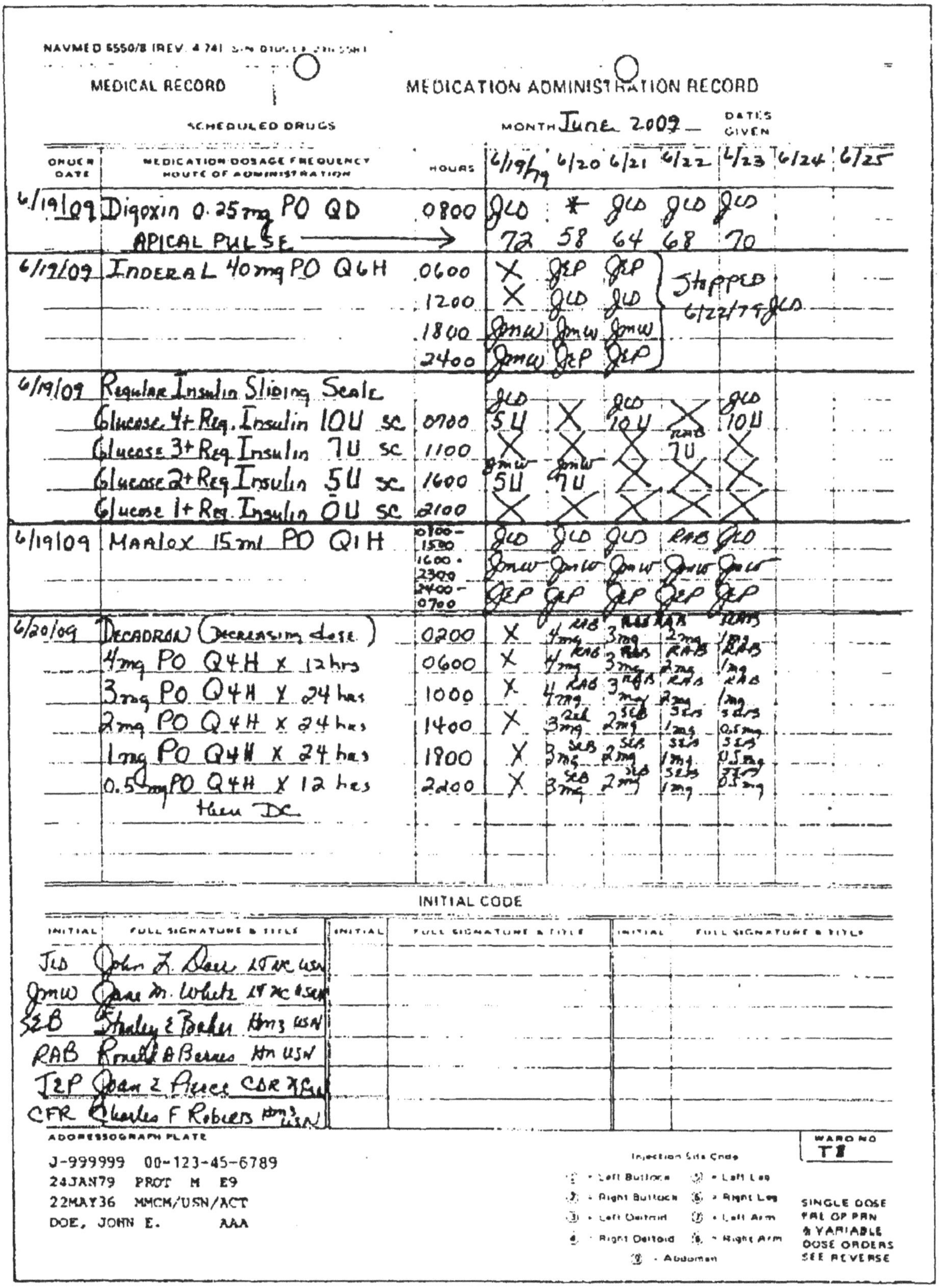

NAVMED 6550/8 (REV. 4-74)

MEDICAL RECORD — MEDICATION ADMINISTRATION RECORD

SCHEDULED DRUGS — MONTH June 2009 — DATES GIVEN

ORDER DATE	MEDICATION-DOSAGE-FREQUENCY ROUTE OF ADMINISTRATION	HOURS	6/19/79	6/20	6/21	6/22	6/23	6/24	6/25
6/19/09	Digoxin 0.25mg PO QD	0800	JLD	*	JLD	JLD	JLD		
	APICAL PULSE →		72	58	64	68	70		
6/19/09	INDERAL 40mg PO Q6H	0600	X	JEP	JEP	STOPPED 6/22/79 JLD			
		1200	X	JLD	JLD				
		1800	JMW	JMW	JMW				
		2400	JMW	JEP	JEP				
6/19/09	Regular Insulin Sliding Scale								
	Glucose 4+ Req. Insulin 10U sc	0700	JLD 5U	X	JLD 10U	X RAB	JLD 10U		
	Glucose 3+ Req Insulin 7U sc	1100	X	X	X	7U	X		
	Glucose 2+ Req Insulin 5U sc	1600	JMW 5U	JMW 7U	X	X	X		
	Glucose 1+ Req. Insulin 0U sc	2100	X	X	X	X	X		
6/19/09	MAALOX 15ml PO Q1H	0700-1500	JLD	JLD	JLD	RAB	JLD		
		1600-2300	JMW	JMW	JMW	JMW	JMW		
		2400-0700	JEP	JEP	JEP	JEP	JEP		
6/20/09	DECADRON (Decreasing dose)	0200	X	4mg RAB	3mg RAB	2mg RAB	1mg SEB		
	4mg PO Q4H x 12hrs	0600	X	4mg RAB	3mg RAB	2mg RAB	1mg RAB		
	3mg PO Q4H x 24 hrs	1000	X	4mg RAB	3mg RAB	2mg RAB	1mg RAB		
	2mg PO Q4H x 24 hrs	1400	X	3mg SEB	2mg SEB	1mg SEB	0.5mg SEB		
	1mg PO Q4H x 24 hrs	1800	X	3mg SEB	2mg SEB	1mg SEB	0.5mg SEB		
	0.5mg PO Q4H x 12 hrs then DC	2200	X	3mg SEB	2mg SEB	1mg	0.5mg		

INITIAL CODE

INITIAL	FULL SIGNATURE & TITLE	INITIAL	FULL SIGNATURE & TITLE	INITIAL	FULL SIGNATURE & TITLE
JLD	John L. Doe LT NC USN				
JMW	Jane M. White LT NC USN				
SEB	Shirley E Baker HM3 USN				
RAB	Ronald A Barnes HN USN				
JEP	Joan E Pierce CDR NC				
CFR	Charles F Roberts HM3 USN				

ADDRESSOGRAPH PLATE

J-999999 00-123-45-6789
24JAN79 PROT M E9
22MAY36 MMCM/USN/ACT
DOE, JOHN E. AAA

WARD NO T1

Injection Site Code
1 = Left Buttock 5 = Left Leg
2 = Right Buttock 6 = Right Leg
3 = Left Deltoid 7 = Left Arm
4 = Right Deltoid 8 = Right Arm
9 = Abdomen

SINGLE DOSE PRE OP PRN & VARIABLE DOSE ORDERS SEE REVERSE

Figure 1. Sample Entries on Medication Administration Record (Front).

MEDICATION ADMINISTRATION RECORD (cont)

PROCEDURE	SPECIAL CONSIDERATIONS
• Transcribe single-order medication, dosage, route of administration, and date and time to be given on back of form. See figure 2 on the following page.	
• After administering medication, initial appropriate block.	
• Transcribe each preoperative (PREOP) medication dosage, and route of administration on succeeding lines.	A bracket may be used to show that all PREOP medications are to be given on the same date and time.
• Enter your initials after administering medications.	
• Transcribe PRN and variable dose medications from doctor's orders to back of form (fig. 2).	
• Enter order date, medication, dosage, frequency, route, and reason for medication.	For variable dose medications, the dosage need not be the same for each entry.
• Enter date, time, dose, and your initials after administering medication.	

NOTE: Some medication orders require modification of basic transcription and charting techniques (fig. 1). These include:

   • increasing or decreasing dose medications
   • medications requiring apical pulse assessment before administration
   • medications administered every other day
   • medications such as insulin administered per sliding scale

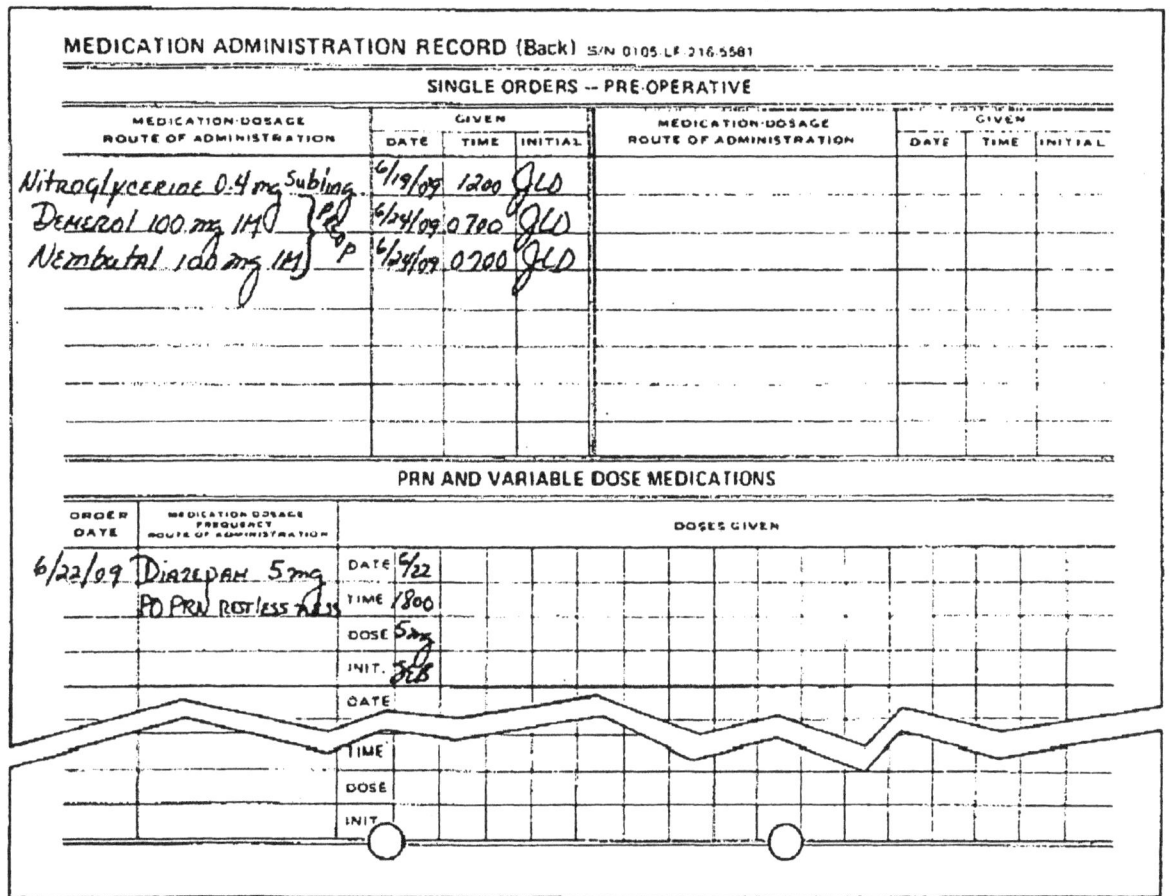

Figure 2. Sample Entries on Medication Administration Record (Back).

III. DROPS
A. Ear

PURPOSE
To instill medication into the auditory canal

PROCEDURE

• See "Guidelines for Medication Administration, General."

• Position patient on side with affected ear upward.

• Clean external auditory canal gently with cotton applicators.

• Straighten auditory canal by gently pulling lobe upward and backward.

SPECIAL CONSIDERATIONS

Patients should have their own properly labeled medication and it should be at room temperature.

Avoid traumatizing when dry-wiping ear canal.

DROPS, EAR (cont)
PROCEDURE

- Instill prescribed number of drops holding dropper nearly horizontally.

- Place cotton loosely in external auditory canal (if ordered).

- Instruct patient to remain in position with treated ear upward for about 5 minutes.

SPECIAL CONSIDERATIONS

Support head as needed. Allow medication to fall to side of canal.

SUPPLIES AND EQUIPMENT

Applicators, cotton tipped   Cotton balls

B. *Eye*
(Ointment Included)

PURPOSE
To apply medication to eye tissue

PROCEDURE

- See "Guidelines for Medication Administration."

- Verify eye to be medicated.

- Tilt patient's head backward and sideways so solution will run away from tear duct.

- Clean eye gently with cotton ball.

- Retract lower lid.

- Instruct patient to look upward.

- Drop medication onto lower lid as shown in figure 3.

SPECIAL CONSIDERATIONS

If both drops and ointment are ordered, instill drops before applying ointment. Patients should have their own properly labeled medication.

Some solutions are toxic if absorbed through the nose or pharynx.

Do not permit dropper or tip of ointment tube to touch the eye. Avoid contaminating medicine container.

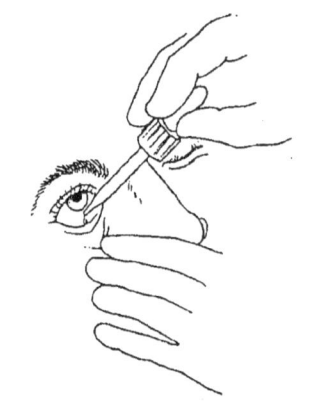

Figure -3. Instilling Eye Drops.

DROPS, EYE (cont)
PROCEDURE
- Apply ointment onto conjunctiva of lower lid as illustrated in figure 4.

- Place dropper in bottle or put cap on ointment tube.

- Instruct patient to close eye.

- Wipe excess medication from inner to outer eye with sterile 2x2s then discard.

SPECIAL CONSIDERATIONS

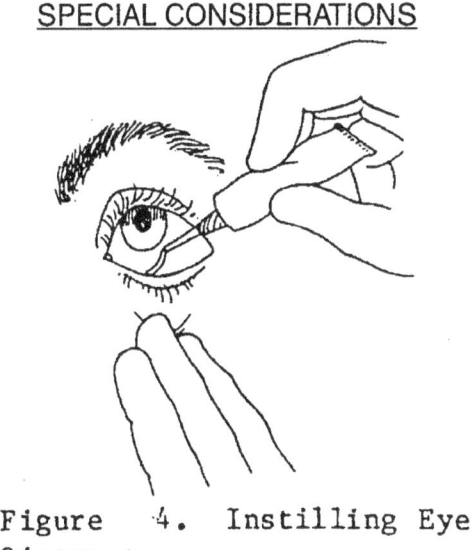

Figure 4. Instilling Eye Ointment.

SUPPLIES AND EQUIPMENT
Cotton balls   Sterile gauze 2x2s

c. Nose

PURPOSE
- To instill medication into the nose

PROCEDURE
- See "Guidelines for Medication Administration."

- Tilt patient's head backwards.

- Fill dropper with medication.

- Instill prescribed dosage into nostril as shown in figure 5.

- Place tissues within easy reach.

- Keep patient in position for about 2 minutes.

SPECIAL CONSIDERATIONS

Patients should have their own properly labeled medication.

Do not permit medication to touch rubber bulb of dropper.

Avoid touching nostril with tip of dropper.

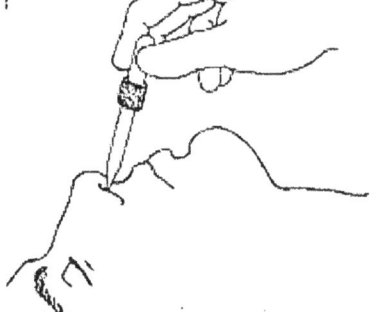

Figure 5. Instilling Nose Drops.

IV. GASTRIC TUBES

PURPOSE
To administer medications into the stomach through a tube

PROCEDURE	SPECIAL CONSIDERATIONS
• See "Guidelines for Medication Administration, General."	
• Crush all tablets and add 30 ml tap water.	
• Assemble equipment and take to bedside.	
• Elevate head of bed unless contraindicated.	Decreases risk of aspiration and regurgitation.
• Expose feeding tube.	
• Place protective pad under tubes.	

• Check stomach tube for correct placement.
   • Aspirate for gastric contents.
   • Listen with stethoscope for air entering stomach as 5 to 10 cc of air is injected into tube.
	Notify physician if tube is not placed properly.

• Attach irrigating syringe to tube with plunger removed.	
• Instill medication into irrigating syringe.	
• Follow medication with 30 ml water and allow to flow by gravity.	Ensures patient receives all medication.
• Clamp tube and cover end for 20 to 30 minutes unless contraindicated.	Allows medicine to be absorbed.
• Reattach tube to suction if indicated.	
• Rinse and clean;syringe with tap water.	
• Return syringe to bedside storage.	
• Record amount of water instilled on I&O worksheet.	
• Record medication administered on MAR.	

GASTRIC TUBES (cont)

Clamp Emesis basin Gauze sponges 4x4

SUPPLIES AND EQUIPMENT

Irrigating syringe, 60 ml Protective pad Rubber band

Sterile dressing (if ordered) Stethoscope Tap water

V. HEPARIN LOCKS

PURPOSE
To administer medications through a heparin lock

PROCEDURE

- See "Guidelines for Medication Administration, General."

- Assemble IV piggyback (IVPB) medication and IV administration set; attach small gauge needle to end of tubing.

- Fill two 2 1/2 ml syringes with 2 ml normal saline.

- Withdraw 0.9 ml normal saline and 0.1 ml heparin 1:1000 into a TB syringe.

- Take equipment to bedside.

- Determine patency of heparin lock.
    - Attach first 2 1/2 ml syringe with saline.
    - Aspirate and observe for blood return.
    - If no blood returns, check for infiltration by slowly injecting small amount of normal saline.
    - If infiltrated, remove heparin lock and insert new one.

- Flush lock with 2 ml normal saline to flush out heparin.

- Attach IVPB medication infusion set to heparin lock.

- Administer medication.

- Flush lock with second syringe of normal saline.

SPECIAL CONSIDERATIONS

Incompatibilities may exist resulting in a precipitate.

HEPARIN LOCKS (cont)
PROCEDURE   SPECIAL CONSIDERATIONS
• Flush lock with heparin solution.

• Record medication given on MAR.

SUPPLIES AND EQUIPMENT

Alcohol sponges Heparin 1:1000	IV administration set IVPB infusion set Needle, 23 ga	Syringes, 2 1/2 ml (2), TB (1)

IV. INJECTIONS
A. *General*

In this section, intramuscular, intradermal, and subcutaneous injections are outlined. Many of the steps are the same for all three methods of injection. Therefore, follow the basic procedure listed below and refer to the specific procedure for special details and equipment.

PROCEDURE

SPECIAL CONSIDERATIONS

•See "Guidelines for Medication Administration, General."

See equipment list of specific procedure.

• Assemble equipment in preparation area.
   • Remove syringe from sterile pack.
   • Loosen the plunger by withdrawing once or twice.
• Assemble syringe and needle.

•Tighten needle.

•Score ampule with file if not prescored.

Prescored ampules are usually indicated by colored ring.

•Clean ampule or vial with antiseptic sponge and break away top of ampule.

•Discard ampule top and sponge.

•Remove needle guard and place on counter for reuse.

• Draw enough air into syringe to equal in volume the dose of medication ordered.

Does not apply to ampules.

INJECTIONS, GENERAL (cont)

PROCEDURE

- Insert needle into medication using aseptic technique. See figure 6.

- Withdraw slightly more medication than required dose.

- Remove needle from ampule or vial.

- Hold syringe and needle vertically.
    - Tap syringe with finger to dislodge air bubbles.
    - Aspirate to clear needle of solution.
    - Push solution up to needle hub.
    - Tip needle and syringe expelling excess solution into sink.
    - Cover and remove used needle.
    - Attach new sterile needle.
    - Read calibrations on syringe barrel at eye level to ensure correct dosage.

- Take syringe and antiseptic sponge to patient's bedside.

- Identify patient.

- Explain procedure to patient.

- Select injection site and position patient accordingly, avoiding undue exposure.

- Clean area with antiseptic sponge.

SPECIAL CONSIDERATIONS

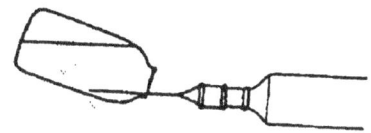

Figure 6. Withdrawing Medication from Ampule.

Do not allow solution to run down shaft of needle.

REFER TO SPECIFIC PROCEDURE: INTRAMUSCULAR, Z-TRACT, INTRADERMAL, INTRAVE-NOUS, SUBCUTANEOUS, OR INSULIN. After performing specific procedure

- Clip off needle and tip of syringe then discard.

14

B. *Intramuscular* (IM)

PURPOSE
To administer <u>sterile</u> medications intramuscularly

PROCEDURE

• See "Injections, General."

• Select injection site. See figure 7.

• Position patient.
   • Place on abdomen "toeing in" for gluteal area.
   • Place on side for ventral gluteal area.

• Clean area with antiseptic sponge.

• Hold tissue taut and insert needle at 90° angle as shown in figure 8.

• Aspirate. If blood appears
   • withdraw needle
   • discard medication
   • prepare new dose
• Inject medication slowly.

• Remove needle quickly while holding skin taut.

• Place antiseptic sponge over injection site exerting slight pressure.

SPECIAL CONSIDERATIONS

Preferred site is the ventral gluteal area.

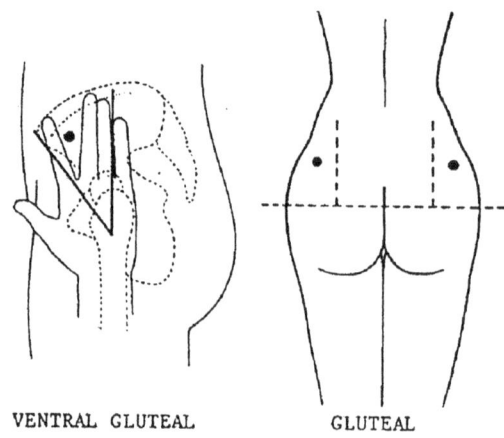

Figure 7. Intramuscular Injection Sites.

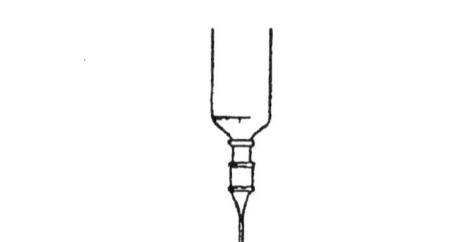

Figure 8. Intramuscular Injection Angle.

SUPPLIES AND EQUIPMENT

Antiseptic sponges (2)	Syringe, 1 to 5 ml	Needle, 21 or 22 ga, 1 1/4 ga

1. Z-Tract

PURPOSE
To prevent backflow of medication from IM injection into subcutaneous tissue

PROCEDURE	SPECIAL CONSIDERATIONS
• See "Injections, General."	
• Position patient.	
• Place on abdomen "toeing in" for gluteal area.	
• Place on back for vastus lateralis area.	
• Place on side for ventral gluteal area.	
• Clean area with antiseptic sponge.	
• Pull skin downward or to the side and insert the needle proximal to midmuscle mass downward at an oblique angle.	
• Insert needle quickly with bevel up.	

• Aspirate. If blood appears
  • withdraw needle
  • discard medication
  • prepare new dose	

• Inject medication slowly and empty syringe completely.	
• Remove needle quickly, holding skin taut.	
• Release skin and wipe area with antiseptic sponge.	

C. *Intradermal* (ID)

PURPOSE
To test for sensitivity to foreign substances

PROCEDURE	SPECIAL CONSIDERATIONS
• See "Injections, General."	Usual dose for ID testing is 0.1 ml or less.
• Select injection site.	
• Clean area with antiseptic sponge.	

INJECTIONS, ID (cont)

PROCEDURE

- Grasp forearm securely on both sides of injection site.
  - Place thumb on one side and forefinger on the other.
  - Hold skin taut.

- Insert needle just under skin surface at a 15° angle with bevel up. See figure 9.

- Inject solution slowly to produce a bubble or wheal.

- Remove needle.

- Read skin test.

SPECIAL CONSIDERATIONS

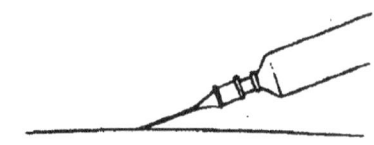

Figure 9. Intradermal Injection Angle.

Do not massage.

Follow local policy.

SUPPLIES AND EQUIPMENT

Antiseptic sponges (2)　　　Needle, 26 or 27 ga, 1 in　　　Syringe, TB

D. *Intravenous Piggyback*
(IVPB)

PURPOSE

To administer medications through an IV line

PROCEDURE

- See "Guidelines for Medication Administration, General."

- Units with IV admixture

  - Check for correctness of medication as in guidelines above.

- Units without IV admixture

  - Prepare medications and draw into syringe.
  - Obtain secondary IV solution ensuring compatibility with medication.
  - Inject medication into secondary IV solution.
    - Label solution with
      - name of medication
      - dosage
      - date
      - time
      - your initials

SPECIAL CONSIDERATIONS

Pharmacy may prepare fluids with added medications.

Do not cover manufacturer's label.

INJECTIONS, IVPB (cont)
PROCEDURE

- Close regulator clamp on IVPB administration set.

- Insert piercing pin through stopper.

- Attach needle to tubing.

- Clear air from tubing and needle.

- Label tubing with
  - date
  - time
  - your initials

- Take equipment to bedside.

- Identify patient as in guidelines above.

- Have secondary IV on standard.
- Clean upper Y-junction on primary IV set with alcohol swab.

- Insert secondary needle into Y.

- Secure needle with tape.

- Open clamp on secondary set and adjust rate.

- Record amount of fluid infused on I&O worksheet.

- Record medication on MAR.

SPECIAL CONSIDERATIONS

Maintain aseptic technique.

Local policy dictates size of needle.

Tubing and needle must be changed every 24 hours.

Primary and secondary IVs. run simultaneously. IVPBs may not run unless primary bottle is lower. It is not necessary to adjust flow rate of primary bottle. It will begin again when IVPB is empty.

SUPPLIES AND EQUIPMENT

Adhesive tape	IV administration set	Label
Alcohol swabs	IV solution (50 to 150 ml)	Needle, 23 to 19 ga

E. *Subcutaneous* (SC)

PURPOSE
To administer medications subcutaneously

PROCEDURE
- See "Injections, General."

- Select injection site. See figure 10.

- Clean area with antiseptic sponge.

- Pinch skin between thumb and forefinger.

- Insert needle at 45° angle with bevel up as shown in figure 11.

- Aspirate. If blood appears
  - withdraw needle
  - discard medication
  - prepare new dose
- Inject medication slowly.

- Withdraw needle quickly.

- Place antiseptic sponge over site and apply gentle pressure.

SPECIAL CONSIDERATIONS

Another acceptable site is the anterior lateral aspect of the thigh.

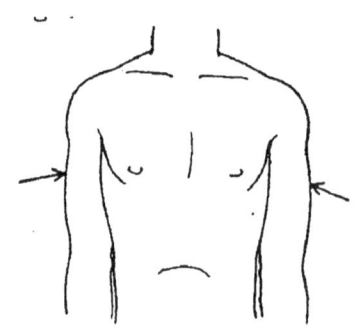

Figure 10. Subcutaneous Injection Site.

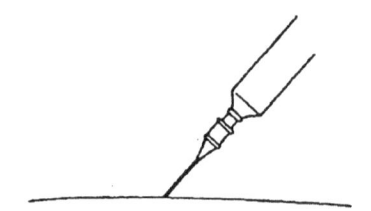

Figure 11. Subcutaneous Injection Angle.

SUPPLIES AND EQUIPMENT

Antiseptic sponges (2) Needle, 23 ga, 3/4 in Syringe, 2 1/2 ml

1. Insulin

PURPOSE
To lower blood sugar

PROCEDURE

- See "Injections, General."

- Roll insulin vial between palms to thoroughly mix and warm.

SPECIAL CONSIDERATIONS

INJECTIONS, SC, Insulin (cont)
PROCEDURE
• Have another person (nurse) check dose you prepare.

• Select injection site. See figure 12.
  • Rotate injection sites systematically as directed by local policy.

• Clean area with antiseptic sponge.

• Pinch skin between thumb and forefinger.

• Insert needle at 45° angle with bevel up (fig. ID.

• Aspirate. If blood appears
  • withdraw needle
  • discard medication
  • prepare new dose

• Inject medication slowly.

• Withdraw needle quickly.

• Place antiseptic sponge over site and apply gentle pressure.

Needle, 23 ga, 3/4 in

SPECIAL CONSIDERATIONS

Do not give to an NPO patient without consulting physician for specific instructions.

Absorption from the arm is more rapid than from the thigh

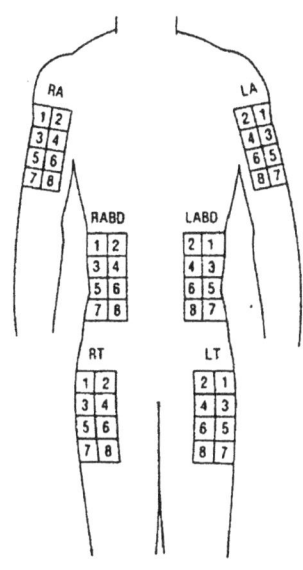

Figure 12. Insulin Injection Sites.

SUPPLIES AND EQUIPMENT
Syringe, insulin

VII. ORAL MEDICATIONS

PURPOSE
To prepare and administer medications orally

PROCEDURE

• See "Guidelines for Medication Administration, General."

SPECIAL CONSIDERATIONS

ORAL MEDICATIONS (cont)
PROCEDURE

SPECIAL CONSIDERATIONS

A. Tablets, Pills, or Capsules

• Instruct patient how to take medication.

For example, if medication is given sublingually, let pill dissolve under toague.

• Check apical pulse rate for 1 full minute before giving cardiotonics.
  Do not give if rate is below 60 per minute.
   • Notify nurse or physician.
   • Record on MAR.

B. Powders

• Remove powdered medications from container with a clean, dry, tongue depressor.

C. Liquids

• Shake medication if it is a precipitate.

• Remove bottle , cap and place on counter inside up.

• Hold bottle with label covered by your palm to prevent soiling label.

• Measure liquids at eye level using calibrated medication cup.

• Wipe rim of bottle before recapping.

• If medication is ordered in drops, count them aloud.

• Dilute irons, acids, and iodides in 120 ml water and have patient drink through straw.
   • Irons and iodides stain teeth.
   •Acids and iodides can irritate mouth.

•Give cough medications after all others are taken.

Do not dilute or give water following liquid cough medications.

VIII. SUPPOSITORIES
A. *Rectal*

PURPOSE
To administer medication rectally

PROCEDURE

• See "Guidelines for Medication Administration, General."

• Screen patient.

• Place patient in left Sim's position.

• Remove protective wrapper from medication.

• Don finger cot or disposable glove.

• Separate buttocks.

• Insert suppository gently through anal opening about 2 inches, using index finger.

• Have patient try to retain suppository for 20 minutes if given to cause bowel movement.

• Hold buttocks together for a minute or two to ensure absorption.

• Remove glove or finger cot and discard.

• Wash your hands.

• Assist patient to a comfortable position as needed.

SPECIAL CONSIDERATIONS

Others can be retained indefinitely.

SUPPLIES AND EQUIPMENT

Finger cot or glove

B. *Urethral*

PURPOSE
To administer medication through the urethra

PROCEDURE
- See "Guidelines for Medication Administration, General."

- Screen patient.

Females

- Place patient on back, legs drawn up and apart, with perineum exposed.

- Remove suppository from wrapper.

- Don disposable glove.

- Separate labia with thumb and forefinger and insert suppository. See figure 13.

- Remove glove and discard.

- Wash your hands.

Males

- Place patient on back with perineum exposed.

- Remove suppository from wrapper.

- Don disposable glove.

- Grasp penis with thumb and forefinger of one hand to expose meatus.

- Insert suppository.

- Remove glove and discard.

- Wash your hands.

SPECIAL CONSIDERATIONS

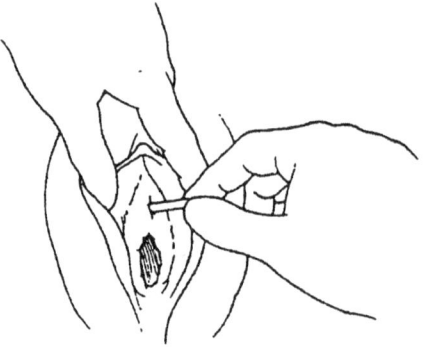

Figure 13. Inserting a Urethral Suppository.

Replace foreskin in uncircum-cised males to prevent constriction.

SUPPLIES AND EQUIPMENT

Glove, disposable

c. Vaginal

PURPOSE
To administer medication vaginally

PROCEDURE,

- See "Guidelines for Medication Administration, General."

- Screen patient.

- Position patient in dorsal lithotomy position and expose perineum.

- Remove suppository from wrapper.

- Don disposable glove.

- Separate labia with thumb and forefinger.

- Insert suppository about 2 inches upward and backward into vagina.

- Remove glove and discard.

- Assist patient to comfortable position as needed.

- Wash your hands.

SPECIAL CONSIDERATIONS

SUPPLIES AND EQUIPMENT

Finger cot or glove

www.ingramcontent.com/pod-product-compliance
Lightning Source LLC
Chambersburg PA
CBHW081822300426
44116CB00014B/2451